ANCIENT LITTLE REMEDIES

Natures Miracle Healing

Rod Stone

Table of Contents

Introduction

As Hippocrates said, "Let your foods be your medicines, and your medicines your food."

From the time of the hunters and gatherers the land has provided not only food but our health needs. Through the regular foods that we eat, but also other plants that grow around us.

If you are living in the United States or a few other areas of the world you would call this history. However, 80% of the world still turns to natural medicine first before they ever consider using a drug or surgery.

Herbal medicine works with the entire body system to help solve the root cause of the illness. Healing is really about self-empowerment.

But, some areas of the world, like the United States has let money control medicine. It all started with John D. Rockefeller who was an oil magnate, etc. in America. He and his friend Andrew Carnegie used the prestigious Carnegie Foundation to change medicine in America and they hoped the world.

The creation of the pharmaceutical industry in the early 1900's forced the change in much of the western medicine. They created a report that talked about the need for revamping and centralizing our medical institutions. Based on this report, more than half of all medical colleges were soon closed.

Homeopathy and natural medicines were mocked and demonized; and doctors were even jailed.

But people are now upset over the high cost of medicine. They wonder why other areas of the world are able to have less expensive medical costs than is found in America.

And more and more people are seeking more natural healing because of the cost and fears of the side effects of drugs from the pharmaceutical industry.

In this book we have created an illness cross reference and a herb guide to try and help you to understand how herbal medicine can provide you with a more natural way to live healthy.

Besides this book you can access our Healthy Living Solutions Book Store to find other useful books to help you enjoy a more naturally, healthy life. Just go to https://products.rhealthylivingsolutions.com/ and if you use the coupon code healthy and you will receive 50% off anything you purchase.

Get a free book every month. Just so to https://rhealthylivingsolutions.com/free-book/ and sign up to receive a free e-book every month.

Origins of Herbal Medicine

Herbs are about as ancient as any existing 'thing.' Dial back the clock 60,000 years, and what information do modern humans have on such a time? Well, we know Paleolithic humans were hunters and gatherers, but farming and modern agriculture were far and away from their minds. Ancient humans ate wild animals, insects, greens, grasses, nuts, and fruits.

There are conflicting opinions on whether or not Paleolithic humans ate more veggies than meat. The region where one lived certainly would play into this.

While nothing is for sure, there is some evidence supporting the idea that humans were using herbs as medicine during these ancient days.

Such an occurrence way back then is not much of a surprise, given that ancient humans had a curiosity that drove us to where we are today, and they depended on their environment far more than modern-day humans.

The Ebers Papyrus

Written around 1500 BCE, the *Ebers Papyrus* listed over 850 herbal medicines. Presented on a clay tablet found in

Ancient Mesopotamia, modern-day Iraq, it seems as if the Ancient Egyptians created the first solid record of herbalism.

You might wonder, *are any of the herbs written down still used today?* Indeed, they are! Aloe vera, basil, belladonna, cardamom, dill, turmeric, and poppy were all featured on the clay for their healing benefits.

Ancient Egypt

It has been recorded that slave workers of ancient Egypt were given portions of garlic on a daily basis in order to help them fight off any infections and fevers that were abundant during those times.

The ancient Egyptians are reputed as being the first civilization to write and make records about herbs and their beneficial properties. There are records dating back to 1500 BC, kept by the priests, who utilized herbal medicines including cinnamon and caraway.

Roman and Greek Origins

As ancient Romans and Greeks invaded other countries, their doctors absorbed knowledge regarding local medicines used in that area. Through their travels, their doctors also introduced the benefits of herbs such as Rosemary and Lavender to other cultures.

Chinese Medicine

Traditional Chinese Medicine also known as TCM, has been around for thousands of years. In this system, the TCM practitioner holds the wrist of their patient in a specific way and feels their pulses. They also inspect the patient's tongue, eyes and skin and then prescribe specific herbs.

Many people who have not had success with Western Medicine procedures have found great relief with this method. Aspects such as Acupuncture, Herbs, and Qi Gong exercises may be employed as part of the TCM protocol. Herbs are the main medicine prescribed.

Celtic Medicine

It is believed that in Scotland and Wales, Celtic Healers and the Druids relied on an oral tradition of herbal medicine knowledge, mixing religion and rituals into the healing process.

British Medicine

In Britain, herbal medicine became abundant with the establishment of numerous monasteries around the country. Herb gardens were grown at each monastery to be used by the monks as well as the local populace.

Native Medicine

Prior to European settlers, local native cultures relied on the plants and animals in their region for their survival. Regardless of the region, the majority of cultures all over the world sourced specific local plants that aided in healing wounds, adding nutrition, and soothing the skin, muscles and bowels.

Of extreme value were antiseptic and cleansing herbs and those which provided a relaxing effect to the system.

Thank you, Hippocrates

Back in the day, a lot of 'doctors' attributed illness and disease to god and superstition. Hippocrates, a Greek physician, thought otherwise and eventually spent two decades in prison due to his disbelief of the practices.

He famously wrote, "Let your foods be your medicines, and your medicines your food." He was *far* ahead of his time, and those who still scoff at herbalism might benefit from reading some of his still relevant thoughts and teachings. From what can be found, Hippocrates seemed to have used numerous herbal remedies in his practices.

Hippocrates used willow bark as a means of lessening fevers and pains. Cut to the 19th century, and scientists used willow to make the now widely used aspirin.

Peak Herbalism Years

The 15th, 16th, and 17th centuries saw the flourishing of herbalism around the globe. Up until this book, herbal writings were primarily in Latin or Greek but were becoming increasingly available as English texts.

Herbalism was never truly an 'elitist' or 'rare' practice and has remained available to all throughout its years of being. In the 1600s, Nicholas Culpeper, an herbalist, botanist, physician, and astrologer, shared herbal medicine with the poor in an attempt to spread medical information to all communities. His peers scoffed at his work, but he continued despite their judgment.

Money Changes

Even though legendary early doctors like Hippocrates, the father of modern medicine, praised these plants as being an innate source of medicine. But what works, works, and the power of these medicines always prevailed and remained our go-to remedy throughout human history—until the early 1900s, when big business in collaboration with the government began to do anything they could to wipe natural medicines off the map.

It all started with John D. Rockefeller who was an oil magnate, etc. in America. His company was Standard Oil, which was later broken up to become Chevron, Exxon, Mobile, etc.

Around 1900 scientists discovered "petrochemicals" and the ability to create all kinds of chemicals from oil. Scientists were discovering various vitamins and guessed that many pharmaceutical drugs could be made from oil.

This was a wonderful opportunity for Rockefeller who saw the ability to monopolize the oil, chemical and the medical industries at the same time!

The best thing about petrochemicals was that everything could be patented and sold for high profits.

But there was one problem with Rockefeller's plan for the medical industry: natural/herbal medicines were very popular in America at that time. Almost half the doctors and medical colleges in the U.S. were practicing holistic medicine, using knowledge from Europe and Native Americans.

Rockefeller, the monopolist, had to figure out a way to get rid of his biggest competition. He went to his buddy Andrew Carnegie – another plutocrat who made his money from monopolizing the steel industry – who devised a scheme. From the prestigious Carnegie Foundation, they sent a man named Abraham Flexner to travel around the country and report on the status of medical colleges and hospitals around the country.

This led to the Flexner Report, which gave birth to the modern medicine as we know it.

Needless to say, the report talked about the need for revamping and centralizing our medical institutions. Based on this report, more than half of all medical colleges were soon closed.

Homeopathy and natural medicines were mocked and demonized; and doctors were even jailed.

In a very short time, medical colleges were all streamlined and homogenized. All the students were learning the same thing, and medicine was all about using patented drugs.

Scientists received huge grants to study how plants cured diseases, but their goal was to first identify which chemicals in the plant were effective, and then recreate a similar chemical – but not identical – in the lab that could be patented.

Although small companies or even individuals conduct some studies about the effectiveness of essential oils and herbal medicine, most are conducted by the food and cosmetic industries. In general, the pharmaceutical industry shows next to no interest in herbal medicine. One can only speculate why, but the industry depends on patented products. You can't stamp a patent on an essential oil.

Since the dawn of time, herbs and specific foods have been utilized by civilizations all over the world for their medicinal properties. Early cultures relied on both ingesting and topically applying plants for their healing properties.

Herbal Medicine in Most of the World

Nick Polizzi in his series Remedy: Ancient Medicine for Modern Illness series stated: "Did you know that 80% of the world still turns to natural medicine first before they ever consider using a drug or surgery? The most used form of this natural medicine by a landslide is herbs. I was stunned to find out that there are green medicines out there that are being used to treat every health challenge known to man from stress and anxiety, to insomnia, to Parkinson's disease, cardiovascular disease, and diabetes, to name a few."

Rosemary Gladstar in the series Remedy: Ancient Medicine for Modern Illness series stated: Healing is really about self-empowerment. No matter what's going on, we use doctors and herbalists, and homeopaths really to help guide us, and to help empower us to make the right decisions. But when we hand over our power to them, we become at the mercy of everything around us, and we're not steering our own boat or reigning our own horses. We flounder that way, I think.

Daniel Vitalis, the host of WildFed in Remedy: Ancient Medicine for Modern Illness stated: "For three-hundred thousand years, we have lived with a diet that contained an herbal medicine component, and for about two hundred years, we have been veering off course. In that time, we have seen a dramatic increase in all of the diseases of civilization, and it's obvious to those people who understand the big picture about what that is. A big component of that, a big pie slice of that, is the lack of herbal medicine, so it is part of our natural diet."

Herbal Medicine today

Herbal medicine works with the entire body system to help solve the root cause of the illness. This is why many remedies may need to be taken for up to 3 months before some people notice a difference.

Of course, depending on the ailment, many people may begin to feel the beneficial effects right away.

There is no miraculous wonder pill with herbs; herein lies the beauty and for some, the frustration. Instead, the whole lifestyle of the patient is taken into consideration prior to an herbal remedy treatment.

This means that during a consultation, not only the presenting symptoms such as headache and fatigue will be discussed.

Diet, sleep patterns, stress factors and bowel habits will all be taken into consideration in order to help paint a complete picture of the patient's problems.

This will allow correct selection of the necessary herbs to enable the body to regain balance and stimulate healing.

Herbal medicine seeks to be holistic, therefore the goal is to treat the cause and not only the symptoms.

The belief is that temporarily curing the body of an ache or pain or illness, but not removing or getting to the root cause, will very likely allow the issue to occur again in the future.

The Four Main Schools of Herbalism

The four main schools of herbalism from which we get herbal remedies and source herbal treatments and preparations are:

- Ayurvedic Medicine

- Traditional Chinese Medicine (TCM)

- Celtic/Roman/European Herbalism

- Native American Medicine

Let's look at each of these in turn.

Ayurvedic Medicine

Ayurvedic medicine has been practiced on the Indian subcontinent for more than 5,000 years. It is a complete system of health and well-being based upon maintaining balance in the body. Part of that maintenance involves using herbs to cleanse, purify and balance the doshas, the elements which are believed to comprise the human body, such as earth, air, fire, and water.

Ayurveda is known as the mother of all medicines because it has served as the foundation for other forms of medicine, including Traditional Chinese Medicine and Western medieval medicine, with its idea of the "humors" in the body, similar to the doshas.

Traditional Chinese Medicine (TCM)

TCM drew its inspiration from Ayurveda, and has been practiced for around 3,500 years. The goal of TCM is to balance the qi, or chi (chee), roughly translated as the life force energy. Balancing and stimulating qi is thought to be the root of health and vitality, and even longevity.

Celtic/Roman/European Herbalism

European herbalism has several strands that date back thousands of years. The Celts, and in particular, the druids, used herbs for healing, religious rituals and more. The Gauls and Germanic tribes would also have used local herbs to treat illness.

Ancient Roman medicine is one of the other foundations of Western medicine. Some texts have come down to us over the centuries that list herbal remedies for a range of purposes.

Herbalism is still very popular in Europe, such as Culpeper's herbs in England or Bach Flower Remedies from Germany. The herbs are usually very pure and often grown organically. Always look for herbs manufactured in the European Union and Britain, or in the US and Canada.

Native American Medicine

Native American medicine has been practiced for thousands of years. It was only with the coming of the Europeans to the Americas that some of their knowledge started to get written down rather than just passed along orally from one medicine wo/man to the next. A growing body of research is starting to show just how effective some herbs can be. The most obvious example is "Jesuit bark" of the cinchona tree, which is the source of quinine to fight malaria.

Some herbalists use all 4 traditions, while others specialize in just one, such as Ayurveda and TCM. It is important to find a skilled practitioner who knows a lot about herbs, and possibly also any condition you might wish to treat.

It is also important to note that just because an herb or spice is natural does not mean it is completely safe or free from side effects. For example, birch bark is the source of the active ingredient in aspirin, but aspirin can kill if you are allergic to it.

A good database should tell you what the herbs are used to treat, and the possible side effects and interactions. On average, a person over 50 will tak8 different medications per day, plus vitamins and herbal supplements. "Polypharmacy" also poses health risks, so be sure to keep an up-to-date list of everything you are taking, and bring it with you to any appointment you might have with a traditional doctor or a herbalist.

Now that you know about the four main schools of herbalism, and the pros and cons of using herbs for healing, let's look next at some of the basic herbs and spices to have on hand at home to treat common ailments.

Illness Reference

Disorder	Herb
Abortifacient (*substance that induces abortion*)	Epazote, Huito, Jackass Bitters, Jackfruit, Loroco, Rosemary, Ubos, Yarrow, Contribo, Cerasee
Abscesses (*a collection of pus*)	Jícaro, Coconut
Aches (*dull pain*)	Pheasant Tail
acid reflux (*stomach acid*)	Santo Domingo, Aloe Vera, China Root
Acne (*pimple*)	Eucalyptus, Linden Flower, Ponderosa Pine, Aloe Vera, Bullhorn Acacia
adaptogen (*helps immune system*)	Holy Basil, Rhodiola, Cordyceps
Addiction (*compulsion for something*)	Mugwort
ADHD (*attention deficit disorder*)	Echinacea, Flax, Jackfruit, St. John's Wort, Trumpet Tree, Valerian
adrenal fatigue (*collection of nonspecific symptoms*)	Nettle
AIDS	Coconut, Noni, American Ginseng
aids digestion	Milk Thistle
Alcoholism (*specific addiction*)	Maracujá
Allergies	Osha Root, Strongback
alterative (*gradually restore proper function*)	Dandelion, China Root, Peruvian Balsam
altitude sickness	Osha Root, Rhodiola

Alzheimer's disease *(type of dementia)*	Nutmeg, Rosemary, Trumpet Tree, Wax Jambu
Amenorrhea *(absence of menstruation)*	Yarrow
Analgesic *(pain relief)*	Dead and Wake Prickle, Florifudia, Guava, Hierba Mora, Holy Basil, Horsetail, Ixbut, Lavender, Man Strength, Maracujá, Mint, Noni, Nutmeg, Oregano, Pheasant Tail, Pleurisy Root, Popcorn Flower, Santa Maria, Strongback, Topa, Trumpet Tree, Ubos, Verbena, Yarrow, Yerba Buena, Yucca, Anamu, Be'o-ja Sacha, Breadfruit, Chichipín, Ciguapate
Anemia *(low red blood cells)*	Chaya, Gumbo-limbo, Huito, Mangosteen, Nettle, Ojushte, American Ginseng, Cacao, China Root, Chipilín, Cordyceps
Anesthetic *(temporary loss of sensation)*	Sangre De Grado
anger	Physic Nut
Anorexia *(loss of appetite)*	Dandelion, Rosemary, Basil
anti-aging	Cypress, Eucalyptus, Guava, Jaboticaba, Macadamia, Ojushte, Pejibaye, Pineapple, Rhodiola, Santa Maria, Yarrow, Capirona, Chaya, Coconut, Cordyceps, Squash Seed
anti-allergen *(helps allergy sufferers)*	Feverfew, Holy Basil, Mangosteen, Nettle, Oregano, Strongback, Yarrow, Breadnut
Antibacterial *(active against bacteria)*	Cypress, Dead and Wake Prickle, Echinacea, Eucalyptus, Guava, Holy Basil, Ixbut, Jackfruit, Lemongrass, Licorice, Limon Indio, Maitake,

Mangosteen, Maracujá, Marañon, Mint, Moho, Moringa, Mugwort, Nutmeg, Oregano, Ponderosa Pine, Rosemary, Sangre De Grado, Santa Maria, Sea Grape, Soursop, St. John's Wort, Sweetsop, Tapaculo, Thyme, Trumpet Tree, Ubos, Venadillo, Verbena, Yarrow, Achiote , Anamu, Anima Ola, Basil, Bay Wiss, Be'o-ja Sacha, Capirona, Ceiba Tree, Cerasee, Cinco Negritos, Coconut, Garlic

Antibiotic *(fights microorganisms)* — Garlic, Goldenseal, Mango Bark, Ponderosa Pine, China Root, Osha Root

Antidepressant *(treats depressive disorder)* — Dead and Wake Prickle, Lavender, Mugwort, Noni, Nutmeg, Popcorn Flower, Pumpkin, Rhodiola, St. John's Wort, Verbena, Yarrow, Ceiba Tree, Coffee

anti-flatulent *(alleviation of gas)* — Ginger, Ajenjo, Epazote

Antifungal *(treats fungal disorder)* — Dead and Wake Prickle, Epazote, Eucalyptus, Garlic, Guava, Hierba Mora, Holy Basil, Horsetail, Ixbut, Jackass Bitters, Lemongrass, Mamey Sapote, Mangosteen, Mint, Moho, Moringa, Mugwort, Myrrh, Oregano, Peruvian Balsam, Popcorn Flower, Pumpkin, Sangre De Grado, Santo Domingo, Sea Grape, St. John's Wort, Strongback, Tapaculo, Trumpet Tree, Anima Ola Barba Del Viejo, Be'o-ja Sacha, Breadfruit, Capirona, Ceiba Tree, Cerasee, Chichipín, Cinco Negritos, Coconut, Copal

Antihemorrhagic *(controls bleeding)*	Cowfoot Vine, Horsetail, Moho, Nettle, Sangre De Grado, Trumpet Tree, Pito, Capirona
anti-inflammatory *(reduces inflammation and swelling)*	Coyol Palm, Cuturro, Dandelion, Echinacea, Epazote, Eucalyptus, Feverfew, Florifudia, Ginger, Gumbo-limbo, Hawthorn, Hierba Mora, Horsetail, Jaboticaba, Jackfruit, Lemongrass, Licorice, Linden Flower, Loquat, Mamey Sapote, Mango Bark, Mangosteen, Maracujá, Moringa, Myrrh, Nettle, Noni, Nopal, Oak, Ojushte, Oregano, Osha Root, Pineapple, Pleurisy Root, Pumpkin Santa Maria, Saw Palmetto, Sea Grape, Soursop, Squash Seed, Strongback, Sweetsop, Thyme, Trumpet Tree, Turmeric, Ubos, Venadillo, Yarrow, Yerba Buena, Yucca, Achiote , Aloe Vera, Anamu, Anima Ola, Barba Del Viejo, Basil, Bay Wiss, Be'o-ja Sacha, Breadfruit, Breadnut, Bullhorn Acacia, Ceiba Tree, Cerasee, Chaya, Chia, Chichipín, Cinco Negritos, Clavel, Cordyceps, Corn
Antimalarial *(prevent or cure malaria)*	Be'o-ja Sacha, Echinacea, Hierba Mora, Jackass Bitters, Marañon, Quebracho Blanco, Santa Maria, Santo Domingo, Venadillo, Ajenjo, Basil, Cerasee, Cinco Negritos
antioxidant *(inhibit oxidation)*	Rhodiola, Santa Maria, Aloe Vera, Capirona, Achiote

Antiparasitic (*treatment of parasitic diseases*)	Florifudia, Guava, Holy Basil, Ixbut, Jackass Bitters, Mango Bark, Moringa, Oregano, Pumpkin, Quebracho Negro, Santa Maria, Soursop, Sweetsop, Achiote , Ajenjo, Anamu, Contribo, Capirona, Cerasee, Chichimora, Chichipín, Copal, Peruvian Balsam
Antiperspirant (*protects against sweating*)	Cypress
Antiseptic (*protects from infection*)	Eucalyptus, Huito, Limon Indio, Mamey Sapote, Mangosteen, Mint, Moho, Myrrh, Sangre De Grado, Santo Domingo, Saw Palmetto, Ubos, Yarrow, Yerba Buena, Ajenjo, Bay Wiss, Cerasee
Antispasmodic (*suppresses muscle spasms*)	Cypress, Dead and Wake Prickle, Eucalyptus, Feverfew, Guava, Holy Basil, Licorice, Linden Flower, Loroco, Mamey Sapote, Maracujá, Mint, Mugwort, Noni, Pheasant Tail, Pleurisy Root, Rue, Santa Maria, Santo Domingo, Soursop, Strongback, Thyme, Tobacco, Trumpet Tree, Ubos, Verbena, Yarrow, Yerba Buena, Ajenjo, American Ginseng, Anamu, Basil, Be'o-ja Sacha, Ceiba Tree, Chichipín, Cinco Negritos, Clavel
Antitumor (*inhibits tumor growth*)	Feverfew, Florifudia, Garlic, Horsetail, Huito, Ixbut, Jaboticaba, Maitake, Mamey Sapote, Mangosteen, Mint, Moho, Sanchezia, Sangre De Grado, Soursop, Tapaculo, Topa, Ubos, Verbena, Yarrow, American Ginseng, Anamu, Cerasee, Cinco Negritos, Coconut

Antivenomous (*inhibits venom*)   Contribo, Coffee, Cuturro, Dead and Wake Prickle, Echinacea, Jackfruit, Osha Root, Rue, Santo Domingo, Anamu, Bullhorn Acacia, Cinco Negritos,

Antiviral *(treats viral infection)*   Echinacea, Eucalyptus, Licorice, Loquat, Mangosteen, Moho, Oregano, Osha Root, Ponderosa Pine, Sangre De Grado, Soursop, Ubos, Barba Del Viejo, Be'o-ja Sacha, Coconut

Anxiety *(intense worry)*   Chamomile, St. John's Wort, Clavel, Dead and Wake Prickle

Aphrodisiac (*increases sex drive)*   Mamey Sapote, Man Strength, Maracujá, Marañon, Nettle, Nutmeg, Rhodiola, Saw Palmetto, Scorpion Tail, Trumpet Tree, Bullhorn Acacia, Cacao, Ceiba Tree, Cerasee, Ciguapate, Cordyceps

Aromatic *(pleasant smell)*   Cypress

Arthritis *(inflammation of joint)*   Ajenjo, Cuturro, Dead and Wake Prickle, Florifudia, Ginger, Horsetail, Inga, Limon Indio, Mamey Sapote, Mangosteen, Noni, Nopal, Nutmeg, Pheasant Tail, Physic Nut, Pineapple, Pumpkin, Sanchezia, Sweetsop, Yerba Buena, Yucca, Be'o-ja Sacha, Black Cohosh, Chaya, Copal, Corn

Asthma *(airways become narrowed)*   Dead and Wake Prickle, Epazote, Eucalyptus, Feverfew, Jaboticaba, Jackfruit, Jícaro, Noni, Ojushte, Oregano, Quebracho Blanco, Saw Palmetto, Sea Almond Tree, Sea Grape, Strongback, Tapaculo, Tobacco, Trumpet Tree, Barba Del Viejo, Breadfruit,

Bullhorn Acacia, Cinco Negritos,
Coconut, Coffee

Astringent *(shrinks tissue)* Cowfoot Vine, Cypress, Flax,
Hawthorn, Huito, Jaboticaba, Limon
Indio, Liver Leaf, Mango Bark,
Myrrh, Orange Jessamine, Popcorn
Flower, Quebracho Negro,
Rosemary, Sangre De Grado,
Scorpion Tail, Sea Grape,
Trumpet Tree, Ubos, Verbena,
Breadfruit, Ceiba Tree,
Chichipín, Corn

Atherosclerosis *(build up* Noni, American Ginseng
in artery wall)

athletes' foot *(fungal* Coconut
infection in foot)

Backache *(soreness in the* Dead and Wake Prickle, Florifudia,
back) Lemongrass, Mint, Pheasant Tail,
Physic Nut, Rue, Strongback, Black
Cohosh

bacterial skin infections Cypress
*(bacterial infection on the
skin)*

Bedwetting *(nighttime* Corn
loss of bladder control)

benign prostate Chichimora, Flax, Nettle, Pumpkin,
hyperplasia *(urination* Saw Palmetto
difficulty)

birth control Barba Del Viejo

black magic Copal
(supernatural power)

Bladder conditions Soursop, Ponderosa Pine

bladder infections	Corn, Pumpkin
bladder stones	Verbena
bleeding	Tapaculo, Yucca, Mango Bark
bleeding gums	Guava
blood clots after childbirth	Man Strength
blood sugar *(if too high)*	Ginseng
blood tonic *(enhances well-being)*	Dandelion, Sangre De Grado
body odor	Limon Indio
boost endocrine *(body messenger system)*	Soursop
boost energy	Ginseng
boost thyroid activity	Soursop
boosts appetite	Saw Palmetto
brighten the mood	Coyol Palm
brittle nails	Horsetail
Bronchitis *(inflammation of bronchial tubes)*	Eucalyptus, Ginger, Inga, Ixbut, Jícaro, Licorice, Mint, Moringa, Oak, Ojushte, Oregano, Saw Palmetto, Thyme, Tobacco, Cordyceps
bruises	Dead and Wake Prickle, Lavender, Maracujá, Pineapple, Peruvian Balsam, Corn, Cypress
burns	Flax, Hierba Mora, Marigold, Noni, Oregano, Peruvian Balsam, Santa Maria, St. John's Wort, Sweetsop, Capirona
cancer	Capirona, Flax, Myrrh, Noni, Pineapple, Rhodiola, Sea Grape, Soursop, Thyme, Venadillo, Wax Jambu, Hyacinth, Anamu, Coffee, Cordyceps, Goldenseal, Peruvian Balsam

Candida *(Yeast infection)* — Echinacea, Eucalyptus, Guava, Ubos, Yarrow, Coconut, Moho

canker sores — Goldenseal

cardiovascular health — Basil

Carminative *(use of herb to prevent gas)* — Ginger, Holy Basil, Lavender, Marigold, Mint, Moho, Mugwort, Nutmeg, Rosemary, Rue, Santo Domingo, Thyme, Yerba Buena, Barba Del Viejo, Basil, Cerasee, China Root, Cinco Negritos

Cataracts *(cloudy lens in eye)* — Noni

Catarrh *(excess mucus in nose or throat)* — Eucalyptus, Huito, Yarrow, Osha Root

Cellulite *(lumpy, dimpled flesh)* — Cypress, Hibiscus

chest congestion — Clavel

chest pain — Venadillo

chicken pox — Barba Del Viejo

chills — Epazote

Cholagogue *(promotes discharge of bile)* — Huito, Trumpet Tree, Yarrow

chronic cough — Saw Palmetto

chronic fatigue syndrome *(profound fatigue)* — Echinacea, Licorice, Maitake, St. John's Wort, Valerian

circulation problems — Noni

cleanses blood — Achiote

colds — Thyme, Wax Jambu, Echinacea, Eucalyptus, Garlic, Ginger, Goldenseal, Gumbo-limbo, Hibiscus, Holy Basil, Mint, Moho, Moringa, Oak, Ojushte, Pineapple, Rhodiola, Tapaculo,

Yerba Buena, Ajenjo, Anamu, Be'o-ja
Sacha, Black Cohosh, Contribo,
Cerasee, Coconut, Cordyceps

cold sores   Goldenseal
Colic *(in babies)*   Ixbut, Licorice, Marañon, Marigold,
                                  Noni, Sea Almond Tree, Sweetsop,
                                  Ubos, Ciguapate
Colitis *(inflammation in   Lemongrass, Pineapple, Sangre De
colon)*   Grado, Aloe Vera

Conjunctivitis *(pink eye)*   Guava, Scorpion Tail, Capirona

Constipation *(bowel   Cuturro, Flax, Goldenseal, Hibiscus,
movement not regular or*   Ixbut, Jackfruit,
easy)   Marigold, Mugwort, Noni, Physic
                                  Nut, Santo Domingo,
                                  Bay Wiss, Black Cohosh, Contribo,
                                  Cerasee, Chichimora,
                                  Coconut
Contraceptive *(for birth*   Ubos, Coffee
control)

controls bleeding after   Ubos
childbirth
coronary heart disease   Wax Jambu
cough   Achiote, Cinco Negritos, Guava,
                                  Hibiscus, Holy Basil,
                                  Jícaro, Licorice, Limon Indio, Liver
                                  Leaf, Maracujá, Marañon, Marigold,
                                  Moho, Oak, Ojushte, Pleurisy Root,
                                  Rosemary, Rue, Sea Almond Tree,
                                  Tapaculo, Ubos, Venadillo, Yerba
                                  Buena, Black Cohosh, Bullhorn
                                  Acacia,
                                  Cerasee, Chaya, Cordyceps, Noni,

cramps	Cuturro, Barba Del Viejo,Cinco Negritos, Ginger, Mint,
Croup *(upper airway infection)*	Oregano, Barba Del Viejo
cystic fibrosis *(hereditary disease affects lungs)*	Cinco Negritos
damaged hair	Coconut
dandruff	Cypress, Florifudia, Goldenseal, Macadamia, Oregano, Rosemary, Yucca, Aloe Vera, Coffee
deafness	Rhodiola, Cinco Negritos
decongest the bladder	Eucalyptus
decongest the kidneys	Eucalyptus
decongest the liver	Eucalyptus
decongestant	Lavender, Linden Flower, Marañon, Mint, Myrrh, Orange Jessamine, Florifudia
delayed menstruation	Epazote, Basil
dental cavities	Copal
dental health	Quebracho Negro
depigmentation *(disease loss of skin color)*	Capirona
depression	Chamomile, Holy Basil, Maracujá, Ajenjo, Basil
dermatitis *(irritation of the skin)*	Copal

Detoxifier *(removal of toxins)*	Jaboticaba, Licorice, Liver Leaf, Strongback, Tapaculo, China Root, Loquat, Squash Seed
diabetes	Breadnut, Coyol Palm, Dandelion, Dead and Wake Prickle, Eucalyptus, Garlic, Hierba Mora, Jackfruit, Maitake, Man Strength, Mango Bark, Milk Thistle, Nettle, Nopal, Ojushte, Rhodiola, Squash Seed, Trumpet Tree, Wax Jambu, Ajenjo, Aloe Vera, Bay Wiss, Breadfruit, Capirona, Ceiba Tree, Cerasee, Chaya, Chia, Coffee, Cordyceps
diaper rash	Lavender, Madre De Cacao, Coconut
Diaphoretic *(inducing perspiration)*	Epazote, Mugwort, Rosemary, Verbena, Anamu, Basil, China Root, Cinco Negritos, Clavel
diarrhea	Corn, Dandelion, Dead and Wake Prickle, Garlic, Guava, Hawthorn, Huito, Inga, Ixbut, Jaboticaba, Linden Flower, Loquat, Mamey Sapote, Mango Bark, Mangosteen, Marañon, Moringa, Mugwort, Nettle, Nutmeg, Oak, Orange Jessamine, Osha Root, Sangre De Grado, Santa Maria, Scorpion Tail, Sea Almond Tree, Sea Grape, Sweetsop, Tapaculo, Thyme, Ubos, Venadillo, Wax Jambu, Anima Ola, Breadfruit, Cinco Negritos, Achiote
difficult labor	Epazote, Feverfew, Noni, Nopal, Rue, Tapaculo, Ginger, Cerasee, Ciguapate
difficult menstruation	Mangosteen

digestive	Turmeric, Ciguapate, Pineapple, Dandelion, Lemongrass, Marañon, Marigold, Nopal, Oak, Popcorn Flower, Rosemary, Santo Domingo, Saw Palmetto, Soursop, Tapaculo, Chamomile, Chaya, Chia, China Root, Moho, Wax Jambu, Ajenjo, Goldenseal, Sea Almond Tree, Jaboticaba
disinfectant	Chia
Diuretic *(promotes urinintation)*	Corn, Coyol Palm, Dandelion, Hawthorn, Hibiscus, Horsetail, Huito, Hyacinth, Licorice, Limon Indio, Linden Flower, Liver Leaf, Maracujá, Marañon, Marigold, Mint, Mugwort, Nettle, Ponderosa Pine, Pumpkin, Saw Palmetto, Scorpion Tail, Strongback, Ubos, Wax Jambu, Yarrow, Achiote, Anima Ola, Bay Wiss, Black Cohosh, Cacao, Ceiba Tree, Chaya, Chichimora, Chichipín, China Root, Ciguapate, Cinco Negritos, Coffee, Peruvian Balsam
dizziness	Feverfew, Guava, Yerba Buena, Cordyceps
drug addiction	Noni
dry eyes	Flax
dry skin	Flax, Macadamia, Aloe Vera
dry socket	Peruvian Balsam
dulled senses	Holy Basil
Dysentery *(Inflammation of the intestines and diarrhea)*	Achiote, Breadnut, Cowfoot Vine, Dead and Wake, Prickle, Epazote, Guava, Hawthorn, Mangosteen, Marañon, Marigold, Orange Jessamine, Pito, Sangre De Grado, Sea Almond Tree, Tapaculo,

American Ginseng,
Cinco Negritos, Copal

ear conditions	Mamey Sapote
ear infection	Moringa
earache	Echinacea, Garlic, Goldenseal, Jícaro, Lavender, Osha Root, Santa Maria, Santo Domingo, Thyme, Basil, Breadfruit, Cinco Negritos, Ginger,
Eczema *(type of dermatitis)*	Goldenseal, Licorice, Verbena,
Edema *(swelling)*	Hawthorn, Inga, Man Strength,
Emetic *(causes vomiting)*	Dead and Wake Prickle, Echinacea, Soursop, Tobacco, Topa, Ceiba Tree
Emmenagogue *(stimulates or increases menstrual flow)*	Cuturro, Feverfew, Guava, Marigold, Mugwort, Myrrh, Noni, Rosemary, Rue, Scorpion Tail, Trumpet Tree, Verbena, Yerba Buena, Ajenjo, Aloe Vera, Anamu, Black Cohosh, Contribo, Cerasee, Chichipín, Yarrow
Emollient *(moisturizer)*	Licorice, Macadamia, Scorpion Tail, Sweetsop, Breadnut, Capirona, Ceiba Tree, Chichipín
emotional stress	Cinco Negritos
enlarged spleen	Breadfruit
epilepsy	Eucalyptus, Mamey Sapote, Maracujá, Mugwort, Rue, Santo Domingo, Be'o-ja Sacha, Cinco Negritos
erectile dysfunction	Venadillo

excess menstrual flow	Hibiscus
exhaustion	Rue, St. John's Wort, Verbena, China Root
Expectorant *(helps bring up mucus)*	Eucalyptus, Hibiscus, Holy Basil, Ixbut, Lemongrass, Licorice, Loquat, Madre De Cacao, Myrrh, Oregano, Osha Root, Pleurisy Root, Rosemary, Saw Palmetto, Thyme, Wax Jambu, Yarrow, Yerba Buena, Barba Del Viejo, Peruvian Balsam
eye conditions	Chia, Madre De Cacao, Mamey Sapote, Sea Almond Tree, Basil
eye infection	Dandelion, Eucalyptus, Goldenseal, Achiote
fainting	Yerba Buena
fatigue	Ceiba Tree, Clavel, Dead and Wake Prickle, Rhodiola, Cordyceps
fear	Cacao
Febrifuge *(reduces fever)*	Ceiba Tree, Copal, Epazote, Florifudia, Garlic, Ginger, Gumbo-limbo, Hierba Mora, Horsetail, Ixbut, Jackfruit, Jícaro, Lemongrass, Limon Indio, Linden Flower, Mango Bark, Marañon, Marigold, Mint, Moringa, Noni, Nopal, Oak, Osha Root, Pleurisy Root, Quebracho Blanco, Santa Maria, Scorpion Tail, Sea Almond Tree, Soursop, Tapaculo, Trumpet Tree, Ubos, Verbena, Wax Jambu, Yerba Buena, Achiote, Ajenjo, Anamu, Anima Ola, Be'o-ja Sacha, Black Cohosh, Cacao, Cerasee, Chia, Chichimora, Chichipín, China Root, Cinco Negritos, Coconut

female hormonal imbalance	Nettle
fertility issues	Mugwort
Fibromyalgia *(Widespread muscle pain and tenderness)*	Mugwort, Rosemary, St. John's Wort, American Ginseng
flu	Eucalyptus, Garlic, Gumbo-limbo, Jícaro, Marigold, Moho, Osha Root, Pleurisy Root, Rhodiola, Wax Jambu, Bay Wiss, Be'o-ja Sacha, Contribo, Cinco Negritos, Coconut, Holy Basil
food poisoning	Licorice
Fractures *(broken bones)*	Sangre De Grado, Horsetail, Trumpet Tree, Breadfruit
Frostbite *(skin and tissue below freeze)*	Peruvian Balsam
fungal skin infections	Cypress
funguses	Copal
gall bladder problems	Verbena, Dandelion, Rosemary
gas	Epazote, Contribo, Goldenseal, oak
gastric ulcers	Moringa, Noni
Gastritis *(inflammation in stomach lining)*	Eucalyptus, Flax, Ginger, Contribo, Cacao
gastrointestinal conditions	Lemongrass, Osha Root, Dead and Wake Prickle
gonorrhea	Bay Wiss, Goldenseal, Huito, Ixbut, Mangosteen, Ubos, Ceiba Tree, Corn
Gout *(form of arthritis, server pain in joints)*	Garlic, Gumbo-limbo, Moringa, Nettle, Pineapple,

	Rosemary, Sweetsop, Cacao, China Root, Coffee, Corn
gum disease	Oregano, Sea Grape, Thyme, Verbena, Goldenseal
gynecological conditions	Black Cohosh
hair loss	Hibiscus, Horsetail, Limon Indio, Mamey Sapote, Nettle, Nopal, Rosemary, Santo Domingo, Yucca, Aloe Vera, Coconut
Halitosis *(bad breath)*	Guava, Limon Indio, Mint, Oregano, Popcorn Flower
hangover	Osha Root, Epazote, Contribo, Corn
hay fever *(seasonal allergy)*	Garlic, Maitake, Pineapple, Goldenseal
head lice	Jackass Bitters
headache	Be'o-ja Sacha, Cowfoot Vine, Cuturro, Ginger, Gumbo-limbo, Hibiscus, Holy Basil, Inga, Lavender, Lemongrass, Limon Indio, Linden Flower, Mamey Sapote, Maracujá, Marigold, Mint, Nopal, Oregano, Pejibaye, Pumpkin, Rosemary, Rue, St. John's Wort, Ubos, Yerba Buena, Yucca, Basil, Black Cohosh, Breadfruit, Bullhorn Acacia, Ceiba Tree, Cerasee, Ciguapate, Clavel, Coffee, Sea Almond Tree
healing after childbirth	Basil
heals wounds	Madre De Cacao, Achiote

heart arrhythmias *(irregular beating)*	Cordyceps
heart disease	Hawthorn, Osha Root, Rhodiola, Sanchezia, Chia, Flax, Garlic, Ginger, Maracujá, Popcorn Flower, Chichipín, Clavel, Coffee, Cordyceps
heart palpitations *(feeling of heart racing)*	Limon Indio, St. John's Wort
heart rate	Tobacco
heart tonic *(strengthens heart)*	Guava
heart weakness	Hibiscus
Heartburn *(discomfort in the upper chest)*	Dandelion, Licorice, Oregano
heavy menstruation	Mango Bark
Hemorrhagic *(bleeding in the brain)*	Dead and Wake Prickle
Hemorrhoids *(Swollen and inflamed veins in the rectum)*	Bay Wiss, Dead and Wake Prickle, Echinacea, Limon Indio, Sangre De Grado, Santo Domingo, St. John's Wort, Aloe Vera, Cacao, Chaya, Peruvian Balsam
Hepatitis *(inflammation of the liver)*	Hierba Mora, Horsetail, Maitake, Milk Thistle, Cinco Negritos, Coconut, Cordyceps, St. John's Wort, Venadillo
Hepatoprotective *(prevents damage to the liver)*	Limon Indio, Liver Leaf, Mint, Moringa, Nutmeg, Rosemary, Tapaculo, Trumpet Tree, Wax Jambu, Yarrow, Achiote, Barba Del Viejo, Ceiba Tree, Chichipín, China Root, Rhodiola
Hernia *(bulging of an organ through an*	Santo Domingo

abnormal opening)	
Herpes *(form of STD)*	Echinacea, Eucalyptus, Holy Basil, Sangre De Grado, Ubos, Aloe Vera, Coconut, Goldenseal
high cholesterol	Flax, Garlic, Ginger, Goldenseal, Hibiscus, Macadamia, Maitake, Mamey Sapote, Mangosteen, Moringa, Myrrh, Nopal, Pumpkin, Rhodiola, Turmeric, Wax Jambu, Yucca, Basil, Be'o-ja Sacha, Cerasee, Chaya, Cordyceps, Achiote, Milk Thistle
HIV *(virus that leads to AIDS)*	American Ginseng, Hyacinth, Maitake, Aloe Vera
hormonal depression	Black Cohosh
hormone imbalance	Nutmeg
hot flashes	Physic Nut
Huntington's disease *(inherited condition in which nerve cells in the brain break down)*	Trumpet Tree
Hypertensive *(high blood pressure)*	Licorice, Coffee
Hypoglycemic *(low blood sugar)*	Barba Del Viejo, Cinco Negritos, Coyol Palm, Garlic, Goldenseal, Guava, Holy Basil, Loquat, Maitake, Marañon, Moringa, Sea Grape, Soursop, Squash Seed, Trumpet Tree, Venadillo, Achiote, Aloe Vera, Anamu, Cerasee

Hypotensive *(lowering of blood pressure)*	Cacao, Dandelion, Dead and Wake Prickle, Flax, Garlic, Ginger, Goldenseal, Guava, Hibiscus, Holy Basil, Horsetail, Jackfruit, Linden Flower, Mamey Sapote, Mango Bark, Mangosteen, Maracujá, Marañon, Moringa, Noni, Nopal, Nutmeg, Pejibaye, Popcorn Flower, Rosemary, Sea Almond Tree, Soursop, Sweetsop, Tapaculo, Tobacco, Trumpet Tree, Ubos, Venadillo, Wax Jambu, Yarrow, Yucca, Achiote, American Ginseng, Anima Ola, Breadfruit, Contribo, Ceiba Tree, Cerasee, Cinco Negritos, Clavel, Maitake
immune system *(body's defense against infections)*	Echinacea, Ginseng , Thyme, Chichipín, Ixbut, Jaboticaba, Jackfruit, Loroco, Maitake, Mamey Sapote, Milk Thistle, Oregano, Pineapple, Pumpkin, Rhodiola, Aloe Vera
Impetigo *(skin infection that causes red sores on the face)*	Copal
Impotence *(or ED)*	Rhodiola, Barba Del Viejo
improves concentration	Thyme
Incense *(when burned release aroma for meditation, etc.)*	Cypress
Incontinence *(Loss of bladder control)*	Physic Nut, Yarrow
increase breast size	Barba Del Viejo
increase strength	Rhodiola

increases nutrient assimilation *(absorption)* — Saw Palmetto

Indecision *(inability to make a decision quickly)* — Holy Basil

Indigestion *(Upper abdominal discomfort)* — Epazote, Lemongrass, Loquat, Mamey Sapote, Mango Bark, Marigold, Mint, Mugwort, Oak, Sweetsop, Contribo

Induces labor — Madre De Cacao, Trumpet Tree, Ubos

infant febrifuge *(reduces fever)* — Coffee

infant malaise *(discomfort)* — Scorpion Tail

infantile catarrh *(mucus discharge)* — Bullhorn Acacia

infantile thrush *(oral fungus)* — Physic Nut

infected insect bites — Achiote

infection — Noni, Jackass Bitters

infectious diarrhea — Goldenseal

infertility — Barba Del Viejo, Feverfew, Sangre De Grado, Be'o-ja Sacha

infertility caused by polycystic ovary syndrome — Maitake

inflamed skin — Chamomile

inflammation — Dead and Wake Prickle, Ginseng , Pheasant Tail

inflammation of the ovaries — Physic Nut

insect bites — Chichipín, Echinacea, Feverfew, Huito, Limon Indio, Marigold, Moringa, Osha Root, Sangre De Grado, Ubos, Yerba Buena, Cinco Negritos, Copal, Marigold, Osha Root

insecticide	Eucalyptus, Jackass Bitters, Lavender, Lemongrass, Madre De Cacao, Rosemary, Soursop, Anamu, Breadnut, Capirona, Cinco Negritos, Hyacinth, Mint, Oregano
insomnia	Chamomile, Cuturro, Dead and Wake Prickle, Florifudia, Hibiscus, Lavender, Limon Indio, Linden Flower, Maracujá, Mugwort, Nutmeg, Valerian, Cordyceps
In place of estrogen replacement therapy	Barba Del Viejo
internal infections	Gumbo-limbo
internal wounds	Cowfoot Vine
intestinal issues	Inga, Sangre De Grado, Tapaculo, oak
intestinal pain	Yucca
intestinal parasites	Basil
irregular menstruation	Mugwort
irritability	Mugwort
irritable bowel syndrome	Mint, Mugwort, St. John's Wort
itching	Verbena
itchy skin	Linden Flower, Oak
Jaundice (*yellow tint in skin*)	Horsetail, Huito, Ajenjo
joint pain	Epazote
kidney conditions	Hawthorn, Nettle, Trumpet Tree, Cordyceps, Black Cohosh, Corn, Ponderosa Pine, Soursop, Aloe Vera
kidney infection	Dandelion, Gumbo-limbo, Pumpkin, Santa Maria
kidney stones	Dead and Wake Prickle, Cacao, Chaya

laryngitis	Lemongrass, Myrrh, Saw Palmetto, Anima Ola
laxative	Dandelion, Huito, Ojushte, Senna, Strongback, Ubos, Ceiba Tree, Chaya
leprosy	Ceiba Tree
lice	Santo Domingo, Sweetsop, Coconut
liver cleanse	Milk Thistle
liver conditions	Licorice, Noni, Aloe Vera, Basil, Corn, Verbena, Eucalyptus, Hierba Mora, Breadfruit, Dandelion
liver pain	Cinco Negritos
loss of memory	Jackfruit
low iron	Jaboticaba
low self-esteem	Cacao
low virility	Cacao
lung congestion	Jícaro, Bullhorn Acacia
lung infections	Ojushte
lung problems	Liver Leaf
Lupus *(autoimmune disease immune system attacks tissues)*	Flax, Licorice
Lyme disease *(tick-borne illness)*	Cordyceps
lymphatic infection *(infection in lymph glands)*	Anima Ola, China Root, Dead and Wake Prickle, Corn
Malaise *(feeling of discomfort)*	Marigold
Malaria *(disease caused by mosquitoes)*	Goldenseal
male impotence	Man Strength, Bullhorn Acacia, Cordyceps, China Root

malicious spirits *(evil spirits)*	Copal
measles	Gumbo-limbo
memory loss	Rhodiola, American Ginseng, Noni, Nutmeg, Rosemary
menopause symptoms	Flax, Clavel
menstrual cramps	Epazote, Chichipín, Ciguapate
menstrual issues	Chichimora, Cerasee
menstrual pain	Lemongrass, Rosemary
mental capacity	Rhodiola
mental fatigue	Cacao
migraine	Eucalyptus, Feverfew, Linden Flower, Noni, St. John's Wort, Trumpet Tree, Yarrow, Echinacea
minor burns	Eucalyptus
minor cuts	Chamomile
minor injuries	Verbena
mood	Chamomile
morning sickness	Lavender, Mint, Barba Del Viejo
motion sickness	Ginger, Lavender, Mint, Sea Almond Tree, Clavel
mouth problems	Sea Almond Tree, Cerasee, Guava, Licorice, Physic Nut, Sangre De Grado, Sea Grape, Yerba Buena
multiple sclerosis	Rue, Trumpet Tree
mumps	Jícaro
muscle cramps	Horsetail
muscle pain	Contribo, Tobacco, Cordyceps
muscle relaxant	Cypress
muscle spasms	Pheasant Tail

nasal polyps	Santo Domingo
nausea	Dandelion, Feverfew, Ginger, Guava, Lemongrass, Limon Indio, Loquat, Mango Bark, Mint, Noni, Sea Grape, Thyme, Yerba Buena, Basil, Chichimora, Cinco Negritos, Clavel
negativity	Santo Domingo
nerve diseases	Hibiscus
nerve pain	St. John's Wort
Nervine *(a tonic calms nerves)*	Chipilín, Cypress, Dead and Wake Prickle, Hibiscus, Hierba Mora, Holy Basil, Jackfruit, Lavender, Linden Flower, Loroco, Maracujá, Mugwort, Nutmeg, Pito, Rosemary, Rue, Sanchezia, Santo Domingo, Saw Palmetto, Soursop, St. John's Wort, Strongback, Tapaculo, Ubos, Verbena, Anamu, Black Cohosh, Chichimora, Clavel, Coffee, Flax
nicotine addiction	Maracujá, Osha Root
nosebleeds	Horsetail
obesity	Dead and Wake Prickle, Flax, Horsetail, Jackfruit, Limon Indio, Loquat, Maitake, Nopal, Pineapple, Chia, Coffee
obsessive-compulsive disorder *(excessive thoughts lead to repetitive behaviors)*	St. John's Wort
oral health conditions	Myrrh
oral infections	Ixbut
Osteoarthritis *(type of arthritis that occurs when*	Flax, Licorice, Nettle

*flexible tissue at the ends
of bones wears down)*

Osteoporosis *(bones become weak and brittle)*	Horsetail, Topa, Black Cohosh
ovarian dysfunction	Cypress
pain relief	Turmeric, Valerian
painful menstruation	Anima Ola, Feverfew, Hibiscus, Licorice, Mint, Sanchezia, Scorpion Tail, Sweetsop, Verbena, Basil
pancreas	Soursop, Aloe Vera, Wax Jambu
paralysis	Pheasant Tail
parasitic skin conditions	Mango Bark
Parkinson's disease *(disorder of the central nervous system)*	Maracujá, Trumpet Tree, Aloe Vera, Clavel
peptic ulcers *(sore in inside lining of stomach)*	Licorice, Sangre De Grado, Ceiba Tree
PMS	Cacao, Nettle, Noni, Rosemary, St. John's Wort, Tobacco, Barba Del Viejo
poisoning	Bullhorn Acacia
polycystic ovary syndrome *(disorder involving infrequent, irregular or prolonged menstrual periods)*	Licorice
poor adrenal function *(physical symptoms of stress)*	Licorice
poor appetite	Cacao
poor brain function	Wax Jambu
poor circulation	Cypress, Hibiscus, Moringa, Nutmeg, Chaya

poor digestion	Flax, Noni, Tobacco
poor immune system	Ginger, Holy Basil, Loquat
poor kidney function	Flax, Ojushte
poor lactation	Dandelion, Ginger, Ixbut, Moringa, Santa Maria, Ubos, Verbena, Black Cohosh, Cacao, Cerasee
poor liver function	Garlic
poor lymphatic flow	Tobacco
poor metabolism	Clavel
poor milk production	Ojushte
poor vision	Chia, Flax, Chaya
postpartum depression	Man Strength
postpartum hemorrhages	Hibiscus
postpartum inflammation	Tapaculo
Preeclampsia *(potentially dangerous pregnancy complication characterized by high blood pressure)*	Garlic
pregnancy tonic *(herbs to improve general health)*	Be'o-ja Sacha
prevent breast cancer	Flax
prevent internal blood clots	Ginger
prevent miscarriages	Hibiscus
prevent prostate cancer	Flax
prevent tooth decay	Anamu
Prevents miscarriages	Barba Del Viejo
promotes dental health	Quebracho Blanco
prostate cancer	Licorice

prostate health — Pineapple, Tapaculo, Achiote, Corn Feverfew

Psoriasis *(red, scaly patches to appear on the skin*

pulmonary emphysema *(disease of respiratory system)* — Cinco Negritos

purgative *(laxative)* — Dead and Wake Prickle, Marañon, Sangre De Grado, Breadfruit, Ceiba Tree, Cerasee

pus-filled sores — Chipilín

radiation exposure — Holy Basil

rashes — Cinco Negritos, Goldenseal, Copal, Mugwort

reduce stress — Ginseng

reduce weight — Chaya, Trumpet Tree

reduces acid — Achiote

reduces nausea — Tobacco

removal of the placenta after childbirth — Jícaro

renal conditions — Horsetail

reproductive conditions in men and women — Saw Palmetto

respiratory conditions — Loquat, Dead and Wake Prickle, Huito, Ixbut, Oregano, Ponderosa Pine, Saw Palmetto, Epazote, Liver Leaf, Cypress

respiratory infection — Holy Basil, Goldenseal, Hierba Mora, Horsetail, Licorice, Osha Root, Pleurisy Root, Santo Domingo, Tobacco, Anamu, Bay Wiss

rheumatism *(inflammation and pain in the joints, muscles)* — Cuturro, Dead and Wake Prickle, Eucalyptus, Florifudia, Garlic, Ginger, Hierba Mora, Inga,

Ixbut, Lemongrass, Limon Indio, Mamey Sapote, Mangosteen, Mint, Nutmeg, Ojushte, Orange Jessamine, Osha Root, Pheasant Tail, Pumpkin, Rosemary, Rue, Sanchezia, Sangre De Grado, Santa Maria, Sea Almond Tree, Sweetsop, Tapaculo, Topa, Trumpet Tree, Verbena, Wax Jambu, Yerba Buena, Yucca, Ajenjo, American Ginseng, Anamu, Bay Wiss, Be'o-ja Sacha, Breadnut, Ceiba Tree, Cerasee, Chichimora, China Root, Cinco Negritos, Copal Feverfew, Flax, Anima Ola

rheumatoid arthritis (chronic inflammatory disorder affecting many joints)

Ringworm *(highly contagious, fungal infection of the skin)*
Goldenseal

Rubefacient *(redness in the skin)*
Eucalyptus, Ponderosa Pine, Rosemary, Rue, Anima Ola

SARS *(contagious and sometimes fatal respiratory illness)*
Coconut

scabies *(contagious, intensely itchy skin condition caused by mites)*
Copal

Sciatica *(Pain radiating along the sciatic nerve)*
Florifudia, Mint, Mugwort, Rue, Breadfruit

seasonal affective disorder *(mood disorder)*
St. John's Wort

Sedative *(promoting calm)*	Cuturro, Dead and Wake Prickle, Epazote, Hierba Mora, Linden Flower, Loquat, Madre De Cacao, Maracujá, Marigold, Myrrh, Noni, Nutmeg, Pito, Popcorn Flower, Soursop, Trumpet Tree, Ubos, Valerian, Ajenjo, Anamu
sexual issues	Ginseng
side effects of chemotherapy	Maitake
sinus decongestant	Eucalyptus
Sinusitis *(infection of nasal passages)*	Dead and Wake Prickle, Echinacea, Garlic, Mint, Contribo, Pineapple, Linden Flower, Oregano, Osha Root
skin conditions	Barba Del Viejo, Capirona, Chichimora, China Root, Coconut, Dead and Wake Prickle, Gumbo-limbo, Hibiscus, Hierba Mora, Horsetail, Ixbut, Jackass Bitters, Jackfruit, Lavender, Limon Indio, Loquat, Madre De Cacao, Mamey Sapote, Man Strength, Moho, Myrrh, Nettle, Nutmeg, Oregano, Osha Root, Pumpkin, Rosemary, Santa Maria, Scorpion Tail, Sea Almond Tree, St. John's Wort, Sweetsop, Tapaculo, Ubos, Venadillo, Wax Jambu, Yarrow, Yucca, Achiote, Be'o-ja Sacha, Cerasee, Chaya, Chia, Chichipín, Clavel, Coffee, Corn, Cuturro, Peruvian Balsam, Florifudia, Breadfruit, Bullhorn Acacia
skin fungus	Ponderosa Pine
skin sores	Guava, Marigold

skin tonic	Cypress
skin ulcers	Huito, Marigold,Nopal
slow labor	Jícaro
smallpox	Noni
smoking cessation	St. John's Wort
soothes membranes	Achiote
Soothes the digestive system	Bay Wiss, Saw Palmetto
sore eyes	Marigold
sore muscles	Basil, Cuturro, Florifudia, Ginger, Inga, Ixbut, Lemongrass, Mamey Sapote, Mangosteen, Mint, Noni, Orange Jessamine, Oregano, Pheasant Tail, Pumpkin, Rosemary, Rue, Sanchezia, Squash Seed, St. John's Wort, Sweetsop, Trumpet Tree, Venadillo, Yerba Buena, Yucca, Bay Wiss, Be'o-ja Sacha, Copal
sore throat	Echinacea, Eucalyptus, Hawthorn, Jaboticaba, Lemongrass, Licorice, Linden Flower, Mint, Myrrh, Osha Root, Pineapple, Sangre De Grado, Sea Grape, Thyme, Trumpet Tree, Ubos, Wax Jambu, Yarrow, Coconut
sores	Jackass Bitters, Noni, Tapaculo, Yucca
spleen conditions	Moringa, Noni, Verbena
sprains	Noni, Pheasant Tail, Breadfruit
stiff muscles	Mugwort

stimulant	Chaya, Ginger, Marañon, Marigold, Mint, Mugwort, Ojushte, Orange Jessamine, Quebracho Blanco, Rhodiola, Rue, Verbena, Yerba Buena, Ajenjo, Cacao, Coffee
stomach conditions	Ajenjo, Aloe Vera, Ixbut, Hibiscus, Limon Indio, Nutmeg, Verbena, Lemongrass, Rue, Goldenseal, Cinco Negritos, Licorice, Pejibaye, Sea Almond Tree, Venadillo, Yerba Buena, Breadfruit, Contribo, Hierba Mora, Huito, Loroco, Man Strength, Mango Bark, Marigold, Mint, Myrrh, Rosemary, Ubos, Yarrow, Yerba Buena, Basil, Chichimora, Chichipín
Stops bleeding from an extracted tooth	Sea Almond Tree
stops menstruation	Popcorn Flower
streptococcus infections *(highly contagious bacterial infection)*	Echinacea
stress	American Ginseng, Cacao
stretch marks	Cacao
strokes	Coffee, Chia
stuffy nose	Goldenseal
sun stroke	Gumbo-limbo
sunburn	Gumbo-limbo, Bay Wiss
sunspots	Pineapple
Suppurative *(fester)*	Chipilín, Hibiscus, Horsetail, Aloe Vera
swelling	Yarrow, Yerba Buena, Achiote

swollen glands	Jackfruit
swollen tonsils	Thyme
symptoms of menopause	Black Cohosh, St. John's Wort, Verbena, Chichimora
syphilis	Echinacea, Mango Bark
throat cancer	Moho
throat problems	Sea Almond Tree
Thrombosis *(blood clot)*	Yarrow
Thrush *(oral fungus)*	Mangosteen, Breadfruit, Coconut
timidity	Cacao
Tinnitus *(ringing in ears)*	Feverfew
tired eyes	Limon Indio, Clavel
Tonic *(for well being)*	Cerasee, Chia, Ginger, Gumbo-limbo, Hawthorn, Holy Basil, Huito, Limon Indio, Man Strength, Mangosteen, Marañon, Mugwort, Nopal, Ojushte, Oregano, Osha Root, Pineapple, Quebracho Blanco, Rosemary, Sanchezia, Sangre De Grado, Saw Palmetto, Ubos, Verbena, Basil, Black Cohosh, Breadnut, Ceiba Tree, China Root, Cinco Negritos, Clavel, Cordyceps, Mint
Tonsillitis *(tonsil inflammation)*	Sangre De Grado
toothache	Breadfruit, Cuturro, Dead and Wake Prickle, Feverfew, Ginger, Mamey Sapote, Nutmeg, Popcorn Flower, Rosemary, Yarrow, Yerba Buena, Cinco Negritos, Coconut

Tourette's syndrome *(nervous system disorder)*   Trumpet Tree

toxicity *(poisonous)*   China Root

Tuberculosis *(infectious bacterial disease in lungs)*   Horsetail, Jícaro, Ojushte, Rhodiola, Topa

Ulcers *(a sore in lining of stomach)*   Eucalyptus, Flax, Florifudia, Goldenseal, Holy Basil, Jackfruit, Mango Bark, Tapaculo, Cinco Negritos

upper respiratory tract infections   Copal

upset stomach   Anima Ola

urinary tract issues   Basil, Barba Del Viejo, Goldenseal, Gumbo-limbo, Horsetail, Man Strength, Mangosteen, Nettle, Nopal, Oregano, Pheasant Tail, Verbena, Dead and Wake Prickle

uterine cancer   Huito, Moho

uterine conditions   Moho, Pleurisy Root, Sangre De Grado, Be'o-ja Sacha

vaginal conditions   Jackass Bitters, Physic Nut, Sangre De Grado, Noni, Dead and Wake Prickle, Flax, Garlic, Hierba Mora, Ubos, Cacao, Goldenseal, Huito

varicose veins *(enlarged veins in legs)*   Cypress, Oregano

venereal disease *(STD)*   Mamey Sapote, Orange Jessamine, Anamu, Hawthorn, Trumpet Tree

Vermicidal *(used to kill worms)*   Madre De Cacao

Vermifuge *(to expel worms)*   Coconut, Epazote, Limon Indio, Maracujá, Ponderosa Pine, Rue, Santo Domingo, Soursop, Squash Seed, Ubos,

Aloe Vera, Capirona

viral infections	Holy Basil
virus early stages	Oregano
vomiting	Feverfew, Guava, Jícaro, Limon Indio, Loquat, Mango Bark, Moho, Mugwort, Rue, Scorpion Tail, Basil, Cinco Negritos
ward off evil eye	Copal
warts	Dandelion, Ixbut
water retention	Strongback
weight loss	Ginseng , Senna
whooping cough	Goldenseal, Saw Palmetto, Thyme, Tobacco, Jícaro
women's health	Basil
wounds	Eucalyptus, Guava, Hierba Mora, Horsetail, Inga, Jackass Bitters, Lavender, Marañon, Marigold, Moho, Moringa, Myrrh, Noni, Nutmeg, Orange Jessamine, Osha Root, Ponderosa Pine, Sangre De Grado, Santo Domingo, Scorpion Tail, Sea Almond Tree, St. John's Wort, Strongback, Verbena, Breadfruit, Capirona, Chichipín, Coffee, Copal, Peruvian Balsam, Goldenseal
wrinkles	Jackfruit
yeast infection *(see candida)*	

Herb Guide

Achiote

Achiote is a shrub or small, woody tree that grows to 30 feet in height and fruits prolifically. It is best known as the source of the natural pigment and flavoring agent annatto, which comes from the orange-red pulp covering the seeds contained within its spine-covered fruits. It is sometimes called "lipstick tree", due to its lipstick-shaped, deep pink or light red flowers.

WHERE IT CAN BE FOUND:

Mexico, Central America, South America, Caribbean, India, Indonesia, Philippines, Southeast Africa, Florida, Hawaii

PROPERTIES AND USE:

Anti-inflammatory, hypotensive, antiparasitic, antibacterial, febrifuge, hepatoprotective, diuretic, hypoglycemic, reduces acid, lowers cholesterol, cleanses blood, soothes membranes, heals wounds and skin conditions, fights free radicals. Treats diarrhea and dysentery, prostate disorders, infected insect bites, swelling, eye infections, cough.

TRADITIONAL PREPARATION:

For diarrhea and dysentery, crush 3 young achiote leaves in 1 glass water, strain, and take in two doses. **For**

swelling, enter a cool herbal bath in which 9 leaves are placed. **For conjunctivitis**, squeeze the juice from fresh leaves directly into the eye. **For inflammation, hypertension, high cholesterol, and prostate disorders**, boil 8 to 10 dried leaves in 1-liter water for 10 minutes. Drink 1 cup three times daily after meals. A decoction of the leaves is used as an antibiotic by the Maya of Honduras and Guatemala.

ACHIOTE OIL
Makes 3/4 cup

The golden oil found in most Latin American pantries is Achiote Oil, which lends a lightly toasted, peppery-sweet depth to rice dishes, sauces, and soups. It's also lovely drizzled on a plate or atop a salad.

INGREDIENTS:

- 2 tablespoons achiote (annatto) seeds

- 3/4 cup extra-virgin olive oil

INSTRUCTIONS:

- Toast the seeds in a small saucepan over low heat for 30 seconds, stirring frequently.

- Add the oil, swirling the pan to disperse the red-orange color, about 2 minutes. Remove from heat and allow to stand for 15 minutes.

- Strain the oil through a fi ne-mesh sieve, discarding the seeds.

- Store in a cool, dark area. The oil should keep for up to 1 year.

USE:

In addition to use in cooking, you may rub Achiote Oil onto skin conditions.

Ajenjo

Known also as wormwood and absinthe, this bitter perennial herb has been used as a medicinal and ceremonial plant since ancient Egyptian times. It is an herbaceous plant with fibrous roots and straight stems. It grows to 4 feet in height and has spirally arranged leaves that are greenish grey on top, and white on the underside. Its flowers are pale yellow and tubular, clustered in ball-shaped heads.

WHERE IT CAN BE FOUND:

Southern Canada, Northern and Central US, Central America, Western South America, Africa, Europe, Mexico, Northern Africa

PROPERTIES AND USE:

Emmenagogue, antiparasitic, antiseptic, antispasmodic, anti-flatulent, febrifuge, antimalarial, sedative, stimulant, and used to treat stomach and digestive disorders, colds, rheumatism, diabetes, jaundice, depression, arthritis

TRADITIONAL PREPARATION:

For all ailments, bring 1 cup water to a boil. Remove from heat and add 1/2 teaspoon dried or 2 tablespoons fresh ajenjo. Allow too steep for 10 minutes. Drink over the course of 30 minutes. Do not use for more than four weeks at a time. **For rheumatism and arthritis**, make a tincture and apply externally on affected joints

AJENJO TINCTURE
Makes 2 cups

Ajenjo has a very bitter flavor that some find unpleasant. Some add peppermint or caraway to mask the flavor.

If you cannot find fresh ajenjo, substitute 1 teaspoon dried. You will need a 16-ounce jar with lid for this recipe.

INGREDIENTS:

- 1 3/4 cups fresh chopped ajenjo

- 2 cups 100-proof vodka

INSTRUCTIONS:

- Pack a jar three-quarters full with fresh ajenjo. Pour in 100-proof vodka to fill the jar.

- Tightly screw on the lid, and place on a windowsill too steep for six weeks.

- After six weeks, store in a cool, dark area. The tincture should keep for up to three years.

USE:

For use as a sedative, place 1 drop under the tongue.

As a digestant, add 10 to 20 drops to an 8-ounce glass of water. Consume 30 minutes before eating.

For rheumatism and arthritis, place a few drops directly onto the affected area, and gently massage into the skin.

Aloe Vera

This small, fleshy herb has appeared in texts throughout recorded history. From a 6,000-year old stone carving in Egypt to ancient Ayurvedic texts in India, a mid-first Century AD Roman text to the Bible, the healing power of Aloe Vera is the stuff of legends. Known in ancient Egypt as "the plant of immortality", it was even given as a burial gift to deceased pharaohs and to Jesus. It grows to about 2 feet in height, with pale green leaves that narrow and have small spines along their margins. Yellow flowers are found on the terminal portions.

WHERE IT CAN BE FOUND:

Mexico, Central America, Caribbean, Australia, South America, Northern Africa, Southern Europe, Texas, China, Florida, Arizona

PROPERTIES AND USE:

Emmenagogue, vermifuge, antioxidant, anti-inflammatory, hypoglycemic, suppurative, boosts the immune system, and treats HIV, skin irritations, diabetes, colitis, herpes, hair loss, acne, hemorrhoids, dandruff, dry skin, acid reflux, Parkinson's disease, and conditions of the liver, pancreas, kidneys, and stomach

TRADITIONAL PREPARATION:

For cold sores and skin disorders, cut open the leaves and scrape out the gel. Apply liberally to affected areas. **For burns**, repeat this process several times throughout the day. **For hair loss**, mash a fresh leaf and apply to the scalp. Cover with a shower cap or plastic wrap and allow to sit for 1 hour. Repeat for 10 days. **For the extraction of deeply embedded slivers**, slice a leaf in half lengthwise, and secure the slimy side to the affected area. Change the leaf once each day for three to five days. **For inflammation, including arthritis pain,**

drink two 6-ounce glasses until the symptoms subside. Do not exceed this dosage. Excessive amounts of *Aloe Vera* taken internally can be harmful.

DID YOU KNOW?

Recent studies indicate that *Aloe Vera's* hypoglycemic properties might make it an important tool in treating diabetes. Several other studies suggest that it might be helpful in the treatment of cancers (particularly leukemia).

American Ginseng

American ginseng's botanical name, Panax, is from the Greek word for panacea, or "all healing". Often referred to as an adaptogen, an herb that helps the body cope with various types of stress, American ginseng has been shown effective in treating a wide array of conditions. The plant has leaves that grow in a circle around a straight stem. It has a yellowish-green, umbrella shaped flower that grows in the center and produces red berries.

WHERE IT CAN BE FOUND:

Minnesota, Wisconsin, Michigan, Missouri, Oklahoma, Arkansas, Indiana, Ohio, Kentucky, Tennessee, Mississippi, Alabama, Georgia, West Virginia, entire East Coast

PROPERTIES AND USE:

Antispasmodic, antitumor, hypotensive, and used to treat stress, anemia, HIV/AIDS, dysentery, rheumatism, fibromyalgia, hardening of the arteries, memory loss

TRADITIONAL PREPARATION:

For all conditions, steam the root for 3 to 5 minutes, until softened. Slice thinly and eat on salad or by itself. You can also eat it raw, though it is woody. **For all ailments**, you may also make a decoction. Boil, covered, a 1-inch piece of American ginseng root in 1-gallon water for 2 hours. Remove from heat, and strain. Drink one-half of the decoction each day for two consecutive days. You can reuse this root. Chop before the second use. **To store ginseng**, pour honey over the sliced roots, and store in an airtight container in the refrigerator.

DID YOU KNOW?

It takes six years of growth before American ginseng is ready for use. It is an endangered plant species.

AMERICAN GINSENG TINCTURE
Makes 3 cups

American Ginseng tinctures are often used by women to increase estrogen levels and alleviate the symptoms associated with menopause. This tincture is also said to be beneficial for people with Type 2 diabetes, helping to lower the blood glucose levels. To make this tincture, you will need a 24-ounce jar with lid for this recipe.

INGREDIENTS:

- 1 cup fresh chopped American ginseng root

- 3 cups 100-proof vodka

INSTRUCTIONS:

- Pack a jar one-third full of fresh American ginseng root. Poor in 100-proof vodka to nearly fill the jar. Tightly screw on the lid, and store in a cool, dark place. Allow to sit for one month, shaking the jar each day.

- Strain through cheesecloth, unbleached hemp, or muslin, and store sealed or in droppers.

Use:

Take 1-4 ml per day on an empty stomach. It is suggested to use for three weeks, and then take one week off.

Anamu

Known in the US as garlic weed, garlic root, or guinea henweed, this deeply rooted perennial shrub grows to 3 feet in height. It has small, greenish-white flowers that appear on thin spikes and rise above its dark green, leathery leaves. Both the root and leaves have a strong garlic-like odor.

WHERE IT CAN BE FOUND:

Mexico, Central America, Caribbean, tropical South America, Western Africa, Texas, Florida

PROPERTIES AND USE:

Analgesic, antibacterial, antitumor, anti-inflammatory, antispasmodic, nervine, febrifuge, hypoglycemic, insecticidal, emmenagogue, sedative, diaphoretic, antiparasitic, antivenomous, and used to treat rheumatism, venereal disease, colds, all forms of cancer, respiratory infections, and to prevent tooth decay

TRADITIONAL PREPARATION:

For all conditions, bring 1-liter water to a boil. Add 1-ounce dried anamu, and boil for 15 minutes. Remove from heat and steep for 10 minutes. Sip 1/4 cup three times per day. **For rheumatism**, grate a 1-inch piece of root. Soak in 1 cup vodka for six weeks. Take a tablespoon each morning. **To prevent tooth decay**, chew the leaves for a half hour each day.

DID YOU KNOW?

Like many other powerful herbs, anamu is used for spiritual purposes, as well. In the Amazon, an herbal bath containing anamu is said to ward off black magic.

Anima Ola

It was on Roatán that we discovered the somewhat unusual medicinal properties of anima ola. Here, Clara Linetnforbs, a bush medicine healer, explained that it's used along with a "half-dead" or dead cockroach and some house paint to remove nails that have been stepped on. Luckily, it's got some other, less strange applications. Anima ola is a small tree of 1 to 10 feet in height. Its leaves are usually broadly ovate-lanceolate, and green with a lighter green or white edge. The margins are serrated.

WHERE IT CAN BE FOUND:

Pacific Islands, Southeast Asia, West Africa, Caribbean, Florida

PROPERTIES AND USE:

Antibacterial, antifungal, diuretic, hypotensive, febrifuge, rubefacient, anti-inflammatory, and heals upset stomach, laryngitis, diarrhea, lymphatic infection, rheumatic arthritis, painful menstruation

TRADITIONAL PREPARATION:

For rheumatic arthritis, heat the leaves over a fi re or in an oven set to low. Wrap the warm leaves on the affected area. The same treatment is used for fevers or to reduce body temperature. **For bacterial infection, fungal infection, water retention, hypertension, upset stomach, laryngitis, diarrhea, and lymphatic infection**, juice the leaves, drinking 1/2 to 1 cup per day until symptoms subside. Mixed with double the amount of water, it is drunk for painful menstruation. **For bacterial and fungal infections on the skin**, chew or mash the leaves, and apply directly to the affected area.

Barba Del Viejo

Barba del viejo, which means "old man's beard" in Spanish, is known by many as wild yam. It is a vine with knotty, tuberous roots. Its thick, green stems are plentiful. Its leaves are red and heart-shaped and turn green when mature. The fruits are dark brown.

WHERE IT CAN BE FOUND:

Mexico, Central America, Caribbean, India, China, Africa, Florida, and other tropical regions around the world

PROPERTIES AND USE:

Antifungal, anti-inflammatory, antiviral, carminative, hepatoprotective, expectorant, hypoglycemic. Used to treat chicken pox and other skin ailments, urinary tract infections, asthma, PMS, cramping, morning sickness, croup, impotency, infertility. Prevents miscarriages. Used instead of traditional estrogen replacement therapy and as birth control. It is also used for cosmetic purposes—to increase breast size.

TRADITIONAL PREPARATION:

For urinary tract infections and kidney issues, boil 3 cups chopped tuber in 3 cups boiling water for 10 minutes; drink three glasses three times per day. **For diabetes**, make the same decoction, but drink before meals. For skin conditions, rub the leaves directly on the skin. **To prevent miscarriage**, boil a small handful of chopped roots with 1-ounce of cinnamon stick in 3 cups water for 10 minutes. Cool, and sip throughout the day for three to seven days.

ROSITA ARVIGO'S BARBA DEL VIEJO TREATMENTS

For Impotency and Infertility:

- Soak 1 cup chopped yam in 1-quart of alcohol for 10 days. Gin is used for men, and anise liqueur for women.

- Take 1 tablespoon three times daily. Cold drinks must be avoided during this time.

FOR INTERNAL HEMORRHAGING:

- Boil 9 small pieces of root in 2 quarts water until reduced to 1 quart. Drink 1/2 glass every half hour until the bleeding stops.

FOR ALL OTHER CONDITIONS:

- Take 1/8 to 1/2 teaspoon fresh or dried root tincture, three to five times per day.

Basil

This spice rack hero packs a serious medicinal punch. Just one-half cup of this highly aromatic, perennial herb contains 97.7% of the recommended daily allowance of vitamin K. Plus it tastes and smells great. Basil grows to 19 inches tall. Its stem, usually square, bears many branches. Leaves are highly aromatic, usually ranging in size from 1/2 to 1 inch in length. Its flowers are green, turning brown when the seed is mature. Basil has been used as a medicinal for thousands of years.

WHERE IT CAN BE FOUND:

Mexico, North America, Central America, South America, tropical Asia, Europe

PROPERTIES AND USE:

There are more than 60 varieties of basil, with health benefits varying slightly by variety. But in general, it is antibacterial, anti-inflammatory, diaphoretic, carminative, antispasmodic, stomachic, tonic, antimalarial, good for cardiovascular health, the eyes, to treat nausea, vomiting, urinary tract ailments, high cholesterol, diseases of the liver, intestinal parasites, earache, headache, depression, anorexia, sore muscles. It is especially helpful for women's health: delaying menstruation, easing the pain of menstruation, and healing after childbirth.

TRADITIONAL PREPARATION:

For fever reduction, nausea, intestinal parasites, and diseases of the liver, boil 2 tablespoons dried basil in 8 ounces water for 2 minutes. Prepare twice per day, and drink while hot. For sore muscles, combine 2 tablespoons dried, chopped basil with 1/4 cup organic olive oil. Smooth on the affected area.

BASIL TEA
Makes 1 cup

Suffering from indigestion, menstrual pain, vomiting, diarrhea, or high cholesterol? This simple tea is for you!

INGREDIENTS:

- 1 tablespoon chopped dry or 3 tablespoons chopped fresh basil

INSTRUCTIONS:

- Pour 1 cup boiling water over the basil.

- Strain, and drink in one serving

USE:

You may drink up to 3 cups per day.

DID YOU KNOW?

Basil is powerful in spiritual healing, as well. Grief, envy, fear, and evil are thought by the Maya to be warded off by carrying a sprig of basil. Those who suspect they are the target of black magic sleep with a bundle under their bed.

Bay Wiss

Also known as briar wiss, bay wiss is a perennial plant with a woody vine that frequently climbs over tall trees. The stems are flexible and thick, and the asymmetrical leaves are oblong, with small flowers that are whitish or yellow green. A large variation of growth in pubescence has led to a number of varieties being named: seasonvine, millionaire vine, princess vine, and curtain ivy.

WHERE IT CAN BE FOUND:

Guatemala, Honduras, Caribbean, Florida, Chile, Mexico, Brazil, Argentina, Colombia, Ecuador

PROPERTIES AND USE:

Antibacterial, diuretic, antiseptic, anti-inflammatory, and treats diabetes, respiratory infections, hemorrhoids, flu, sore muscles, constipation, gonorrhea. Soothes the digestive system, rheumatism, sunburns.

TRADITIONAL PREPARATION:

For rheumatism and hemorrhoids, make an infusion by boiling 1 large handful bay wiss vine in 1-gallon water. Drink three times per day. **For sore muscles**, coat sun-warmed leaves with almond oil, and apply directly to the affected area. Leaves can be made into poultices to **reduce inflammation** and are sometimes used after childbirth. A flower decoction can be used as an antiseptic **to disinfect and wash wounds**, as well as to soothe sunburned skin. Berries can be fermented in a beverage, which is good to drink **as a laxative and as a diuretic**.

DID YOU KNOW?

Bay wiss often grows aerial roots, which is how it gained the name curtain ivy. Speculation is that the roots grow in an aerial manner to access additional water resources. The roots grow very fast, at an approximate rate of 1 inch every 3 hours.

Be'o-ja Sacha

Also known as *ajo sacha*, or false garlic, this evergreen shrub or vine is native to the Amazon. It has bright green leaves that grow to 6 inches and flowers that are purple to white in color. It is often administered during ayahuasca ceremonies and used to ward off evil.

WHERE IT CAN BE FOUND:

Amazon rainforest, Central America

PROPERTIES AND USE:

Analgesic, anti-inflammatory, febrifuge, antispasmodic, antiviral, antifungal, antibacterial, antimalarial. Used as a pregnancy tonic, and treats high cholesterol, colds, flu, epilepsy, uterine conditions, skin conditions, arthritis, sore muscles, rheumatism, infertility, and headache.

TRADITIONAL PREPARATION:

To make a decoction, boil a few large leaves in 1-gallon water for 30 minutes. Steep for 30 minutes. **For skin**

conditions, arthritis, sore muscles, and rheumatism, use the bark as a poultice. It is also available in tincture and capsule form.

Black Cohosh

Black cohosh, a member of the buttercup family, is a hearty, herbaceous perennial of up to 8 feet tall, with a long plume of white flowers at the top and leaves that are irregular and serrated on the edges. The root is black when harvested in the fall. *Black cohosh* has for centuries been used medicinally by Native Americans. Today, it is used to treat menopause.

WHERE IT CAN BE FOUND:

Quebec, Canada; Ontario, Canada; Iowa; Missouri; Arkansas; and east of the Mississippi, excluding Wisconsin, Louisiana, Massachusetts, Rhode Island

PROPERTIES AND USE:

Emmenagogue, nervine, tonic, febrifuge, diuretic, and used to treat headache, colds, cough, constipation, backache, gynecological conditions, kidney disorders, poor lactation, hormonal depression, arthritis, osteoporosis, symptoms of menopause

TRADITIONAL PREPARATION:

For all conditions, boil a small handful of chopped roots in 1-gallon water for 30 minutes. Remove from heat and allow to steep an additional 30 minutes. Strain, and sip a cup per day. You may wish to add a small amount of ginger to improve the infusion's strong flavor.

Breadfruit

This tree grows up to 60 feet tall and has diagonal branches and dark-green lobed leaves. The lime-green, prickly, globular fruits weigh up to 10 pounds each. A good source of iron, calcium, niacin, potassium, riboflavin, and amino acids, it is an important foodstuff. Like the banana and plantain, it is eaten ripe as a "fruit" or unripe as a vegetable.

WHERE IT CAN BE FOUND:

Pacific Islands, Southeast Asia, New Guinea, Caribbean, Africa

PROPERTIES AND USE:

Analgesic, antifungal, astringent, purgative, hypotensive, anti-inflammatory, and treats diarrhea, stomachache, liver disease, diabetes, thrush, earache, enlarged spleen, headache, asthma, wounds, broken bones, sprains, skin infections, sciatica, toothache

TRADITIONAL PREPARATION:

For headaches, broken bones, sprains, and skin infections, slightly crush the leaves, and place directly on the affected area. For thrush, crushed leaves are applied directly on the tongue or are chewed. **For earaches**, squeeze the juice from the leaves, and drop into the ear. **For an enlarged spleen**, roast the leaves and then crush into a powder. Use 1 teaspoon in 2 cups boiling water and repeat twice per day. This same powder is applied directly on the gums for toothaches. **For sciatica**, press latex from the leaves, and place into a compress that is bandaged directly onto the spine. This procedure can also be used for skin conditions and wounds. One tablespoon latex diluted in water is used to treat diarrhea. **For hypertension**, crush 1 yellowing leaf and boil in 2 cups water. Cool. Sip throughout the day. In the Pacific Islands, the bark is used in a decoction for headaches. In the West Indies, a decoction is used to control diabetes. **For broken bones or sprains**, massage the latex directly on the affected area.

Breadnut

Breadnut is a single-stemmed evergreen tree that grows to 50 feet or more and has a spreading canopy of large, alternating leaves and buttresses at the base. The roots spread and grow on or slightly below the surface. Fruit is a fleshy oval 5 to 8 inches long, with dull green to yellow-green skin and a spiny texture. It is an important source of nutrition, as it's a good source of potassium, phosphorus, calcium, and iron. Breadnut fruit tincture is a popular tonic in Jamaica.

WHERE IT CAN BE FOUND:

Caribbean, Central America, tropical South America, New Guinea, Southeast Asia, coastal West Africa, Tahiti, Indonesia, Hawaii

PROPERTIES AND USE:

Emollient, anti-inflammatory, anti-allergen, tonic, insecticidal, and treats dysentery, rheumatism, diabetes

TRADITIONAL PREPARATION:

To repel mosquitos, sand fleas, and gnats, burn the male flowers. You may also rub this on the skin. For diabetes, macerate 3 leaves in 2 cups water and sip throughout the day. **For rheumatism**, add 9 leaves to a cool bath.

DID YOU KNOW?

Is that a breadnut, breadfruit, or jackfruit? Breadnut fruits can be distinguished from its close relative the breadfruit by its very spiny fruits with little pulp and many large, light-brown seeds that comprise 30 – 50% of its weight. The breadfruit is seedless. Jackfruit, another relative, has larger fruit and smaller leaves without lobes.

Bullhorn Acacia

Also known as cockspur, bullhorn acacia gets its name from the enlarged, hollow stipular spines that occur in pairs at the base of leaves and resemble steer horns. It is a small tree that grows to 20 feet tall.

WHERE IT CAN BE FOUND:

Mexico, Central America, Western India, Bangladesh, Florida, West Indies

PROPERTIES AND USE:

Antivenomous, anti-inflammatory, aphrodisiac, and treats male impotence, infantile catarrh, asthma, cough, lung congestion, poisoning, headache, acne, inflammation of the skin

TRADITIONAL PREPARATION:

For acne and inflammation of the skin, boil a 1-inch by 10-inch piece of bark in 1-gallon water. Cool, and use as a wash for the affected area. **For impotence**, boil 1-inch by 6-inch strip of bark in 3 cups water for 10 minutes, drinking before meals for 7 days. **For asthma, congestion, coughs, headaches, and poisoning**, boil 9 thorns in 3 cups water for 10 minutes. Drink 2 cups throughout the day. **For snakebites**, chew on a strip of bark, swallowing the juices, then apply the remaining fiber as a poultice on the bite.

DID YOU KNOW?

Throughout Central America, the symbiotic relationship between the aggressive acacia ant (*Pseudomyrmex ferruginea*) and the bullhorn acacia is famous. The ants live in the bullhorn acacia's thorns, emerging to attack other plants, insects, humans, and animals that come in contact with the tree.

Cacao

Native to Mesoamerica, the cacao tree is a small evergreen that typically grows to only 40 feet. It has small, white flowers and a football-shaped fruit, a cacao pod, that contains 40 to 60 seeds. The fat from these seeds is the source of cocoa butter. Raw cacao has recently been recognized as a superfood, something the ancient Maya knew 2,000 years ago. Cacao was a popular tonic for the royals, part of every one of their ceremonies, and was immortalized in their art.

WHERE IT CAN BE FOUND:

Mexico, Central America, South America

PROPERTIES AND USE:

Stimulant, diuretic, febrifuge, aphrodisiac, hypotensive, and used to treat, anemia, poor appetite, mental fatigue, poor lactation, kidney stones, low virility, gout, hemorrhoids, gastritis, stress, low self-esteem, fear, timidity. It alleviates mental fatigue and PMS and treats vaginal irritation and stretch marks.

TRADITIONAL PREPARATION:

To soothe the skin, create a salve with equal parts cocoa butter and sesame or almond oil. Apply directly on the skin. This is also great for cracked lips, and on the hands and feet. **For hypertension and as a diuretic**, place 2 fresh leaves in 2 cups boiling water. Drink in one sitting. **For hemorrhoids or vaginal irritation**, make suppositories with 3 parts cacao butter to 1-part almond oil. Blend, and place it in plastic wrap. Shape it into the appropriate size and shape, and chill it for 1 hour. Remove from plastic wrap and insert into the anus or vagina. **For low self-esteem, fear, and timidity**, eat 1 cacao bean or 1/2-ounce dark chocolate (at least 70% cacao) 30 minutes prior to entering a stressful situation, meeting, or encounter.

MAYA CACAO - DRINK OF THE GODS

This recipe, ancient in origin, is not the sweet hot chocolate with which most are familiar. It is used at modern-day ceremonies—weddings, birthdays, anniversaries—and is great to treat both coughs and gastritis. For authenticity, use unsweetened Maya cacao crafted in Mexico or Honduras. The red chili is what gives this drink its characteristic flavor. Give it a try!

INGREDIENTS:

- 3 cups water

- 1 to 2 cinnamon sticks

- 8 ounces bittersweet Maya chocolate paste (or 3 tablets Mexican unsweetened chocolate, cut into small pieces)

- 2 tablespoons wild pure honey or raw sugar to taste

- 1 pinch of dried red chili

- 1 dried organic grown vanilla bean, split lengthwise

- 1 tablespoon roasted peanuts, ground extra fine (this Aztec ingredient is optional)

INSTRUCTIONS:

- In a large saucepan over medium-high heat, bring the water to a boil.

- Add the cinnamon sticks and cook until the liquid is reduced to 2 1/2 cups.

- Remove the cinnamon sticks; add the vanilla bean and lower the heat to medium.

- Wait until bubbles appear around the edge, and then reduce the heat to low. Add the chocolate pieces and honey. Optionally, add the ground peanuts.

- Mix well and whisk occasionally until chocolate is melted.

- Turn off heat and remove vanilla bean. Whisk vigorously to create a light foam effect.

- Sprinkle with the dried chili pepper and serve.

USE:

If you used peanuts in the recipe, sprinkle a bit more on top. Milk is not traditionally used, but you may add some to taste.

Capirona

This tree grows to 100 feet and has light green bark in youth, dark brown bark in maturity. The bark sheds periodically and is harvested for medicine. The upper branches create a large canopy. It originates from the Amazon Basin and is an admixture used in ayahuasca rituals.

WHERE IT CAN BE FOUND:

Bolivia, Brazil, Colombia, Ecuador, Peru

PROPERTIES AND USE:

Antibacterial, antifungal, antioxidant, anti-aging, insecticidal, emollient, antiparasitic, antihemorrhagic, vermifuge, and used to treat skin conditions including depigmentation, wounds, burns, conjunctivitis, diabetes, cancer

TRADITIONAL PREPARATION:

To treat diabetes, 2 pounds bark is boiled in 2.5 gallons water until 1-gallon remains. Five ounces are drunk per day. This bark decoction is also used for **conjunctivitis and fungal infections of the skin**. A bark poultice is made **for wounds and burns**.

Ceiba Tree

Also known as *kapok* or silk cotton tree, Ceiba is the sacred tree of the Maya. It is said to unite all three realms, with its branches reaching up into the upperworld, its roots reaching into the underworld, and its trunk connecting the two in the earth plane. It is a massive tree up to 230 feet tall, with a straight, branchless, cylindrical trunk, and huge, spreading canopy. It has buttress roots, and fruit in an oblong-ellipsoid shape. The fruit contains seeds and a mass of white or greyish floss.

WHERE IT CAN BE FOUND:

Mexico, Central America, South America, Indonesia, Philippines, West Africa, Cambodia, South Florida

PROPERTIES AND USE:

Hepatoprotective, hypotensive, antidepressant, diuretic, emetic, purgative, aphrodisiac, tonic, laxative, astringent, purgative, antibacterial, antifungal, laxative, anti-inflammatory, emollient, antispasmodic, febrifuge. Treats gonorrhea, headache, peptic ulcers, rheumatism, leprosy, diabetes, and fatigue.

TRADITIONAL PREPARATION:

For headaches, apply the leaves directly on the forehead. **For diabetes and depression**, boil a 1-inch by 10-inch strip of bark in 1-gallon water. Cool, and sip throughout the day. **As a laxative**, boil a large handful of leaves in 2 cups water. Strain, and drink warm.

DID YOU KNOW?

Clinical trials suggest that Ceiba seed oil might be effective in preventing heart disease and cancer.

Cerasee

This herbaceous vine grows to 6 feet tall and has a delicate stem from which many branches and coiled tendrils grow. The alternating leaves are deeply lobed, and its flowers are yellow. The fruits, which emerge as green, turn yellow orange when mature. The seeds are covered in a bright-red pulp. Also known as bitter melon, bitter gourd, bitter squash, *sorosi, goya, pare*, balsam pear, and *condiamor*. Next to marijuana, it is the most medicinal plant in Jamaica, where bush medicine still thrives today.

WHERE IT CAN BE FOUND:

Asia, Central America, Amazon, Caribbean, Japan, Pacific Islands, Africa, Alabama, Connecticut, Florida, Hawaii, Kentucky, Louisiana, Pennsylvania, Texas

PROPERTIES AND USE:

Antibacterial, antitumor, hypotensive, febrifuge, abortifacient, emmenagogue, hypoglycemic, anti-inflammatory, aphrodisiac, antifungal, antiparasitic, antimalarial, carminative, purgative, antiseptic, tonic. Treats high cholesterol, diabetes, rheumatism, difficult labor, poor lactation, menstrual issues, skin conditions, colds, cough, headache, constipation, mouth sores.

TRADITIONAL PREPARATION:

For skin conditions, boil a large handful of the leaves and vine in 1-gallon water. Allow to sit for 30 minutes. Strain, and allow to cool. Wash the affected area with the decoction. **For**

rashes, place 9 leaves in a cool bath. You may wish to add in a small handful of quaco bush (Mikania micrantha). **For all other conditions**, boil a small handful of leaves and vine in 3 cups water for 10 minutes. Repeat daily for up to 10 days. **For mouth sores**, chew the leaves.

Chamomile

Chamomile is an herb that comes from the daisy-like flowers of the Asteraceae plant family. It has been consumed for centuries as a natural remedy for several health conditions.

WHERE IT CAN BE FOUND:

Western Europe, India and western Asia. It escaped cultivation and grows abundant throughout the United States.

PROPERTIES AND USE:

Mood disorders, digestive issues, help relieve depression, anxiety, sleep issues. Can be used for minor cuts and abrasions, and to soothe inflamed skin.

TRADITIONAL PREPARATION:

A cup of chamomile tea is a soothing swap for regular tea or coffee, and ideal after meals or before bed.

Chaya

This shrub of 10 to 16 feet tall is often called tree spinach. It has broad leaves comprised of three or more lobes with fleshly pentioles. Its white-colored flowers may contain three-forked arrangements. Chaya is richer in iron than spinach, and is an important source of potassium, protein, vitamins A and C, calcium, iron, phosphorus, niacin, riboflavin, and thiamine. Do not eat the leaves raw, as they contain hydrocyanic glucosides. Cooking deactivates the toxicity. Do not prepare in aluminum, as it can cause a toxic reaction. It is known as *chatate* in Honduras and *chicasquil* in Costa Rica.

WHERE IT CAN BE FOUND:

Mexico, Central America, Southern Texas, Florida

PROPERTIES AND USE:

Digestive, laxative, diuretic, anti-inflammatory, anti-aging, stimulant. Used to treat poor circulation, poor vision, high cholesterol, cough, arthritis, diabetes, hemorrhoids, kidney stones, skin conditions, anemia. Helps reduce weight.

TRADITIONAL PREPARATION:

For all conditions, boil 2 teaspoons chopped fresh Chaya leaves in 1-liter water for 30 minutes. Strain, and sip throughout the day. **For skin conditions**, use the cooled decoction as a wash on the affected area. **For weight loss or general conditions**, pour 1-liter water in a glass container with lid. Add four medium-sized leaves. Place in the sun for two hours, and then serve over ice before meals. You may wish to add fresh mint for flavor and lemon to detoxify your system.

Chia

Annual herb growing to 2 1/2 feet by 2 feet, with opposite leaves and white or purple flowers. The seeds are small, dark ovals of .039 inches that develop a gel-like coating when soaked. A superfood, chia is rich in niacin, thiamine, zinc, calcium, manganese, protein, and easily digested fats. The ancient Aztec and Maya consumed it before battle and on long journeys.

WHERE IT CAN BE FOUND:

Central America, Mexico, Arizona, California, New Mexico, Nevada, Utah

PROPERTIES AND USE:

Digestive, disinfectant, febrifuge, anti-inflammatory, tonic. Used to treat stroke, heart conditions, obesity, diabetes, skin conditions, and eye conditions including poor vision.

TRADITIONAL PREPARATION:

For all conditions, combine 2 tablespoons chia seeds with 1 glass room-temperature water. Drink in one sitting. **For weight loss**, combine 1 tablespoon chia seeds in 2 ounces water, coconut water, or unsweetened cranberry juice. Allow to sit for 10 minutes. Drink 30 minutes before breakfast. **For skin conditions**, combine 2 tablespoons chia seeds with 4 ounces water. Allow to sit for at least 30 minutes or overnight. Apply the gelatinous mixture to the affected area.

DID YOU KNOW?

Pack chia next time you travel to ward off jet lag. This tiny seed contains tryptophan, which can help regulate our sleep-wake cycle when traveling.

Chichimora

This plant in the curcubit (*Cucurbitaceae*), or gourd, family has reddish stems and alternating leaves. Its flowers are yellow or orange, and the spherical fruit can grow to 2 pounds. It is high in amino acids, linoleic acid, vitamins A and B, and several minerals. The seeds are used for women's medicine and digestive issues.

WHERE IT CAN BE FOUND:

Central America to Brazil, Caribbean

PROPERTIES AND USE:

Stomachic, diuretic, nervine, antiparasitic, febrifuge, and used to treat rheumatism, constipation, nausea, symptoms of menopause, menstrual difficulties, benign prostate hyperplasia, skin conditions

TRADITIONAL PREPARATION:

For all conditions, boil a large handful of the chopped root in 1-liter water for 30 minutes. Remove from heat and allow too steep for 30 minutes. Strain, and sip throughout the day. **For women's issues**, boil 1-gallon water. Remove from heat. Add 1/2 cup seeds and allow too steep for 15 minutes. Strain, and allow to cool. Sip three glasses per day. This same infusion is used for digestive issues. Sip the liquid throughout the day. **For skin conditions**, scoop out the fruit's pulpy insides, and apply directly onto the affected area. For fevers, place the fruit's skin directly on the forehead.

Chichipín

This semi-woody shrub grows to 9 feet tall, and has deeply veined, red-tinted leaves. Its flowers are bright orange-red and tubular. The fruit is a red berry that turns black when ripe. It is known as Polly red head, red head, scarletbush, firebush, and *sanalo-todo*. Its name in Mopan Maya is *Ix-canan*, which means "guardian of the forest". On the Caribbean island of Roatán, it is known as healin' draw.

WHERE IT CAN BE FOUND:

Mexico, Caribbean, Central America, South America, Florida

PROPERTIES AND USE:

Anti-inflammatory, astringent, emmenagogue, emollient, stomachic, analgesic, febrifuge, diuretic, antifungal, antiparasitic, antispasmodic, hepatoprotective, and is used to treat heart disease, menstrual cramps, wounds, skin conditions, and insect bites. It enhances immunity.

TRADITIONAL PREPARATION:

For skin conditions, fungus, and insect bites, boil 2 large handfuls of flowers, leaves, and stems in 2 gallons water for 10 minutes. Wash the affected area with the warm liquid or use as a bath. **For sores and ulcers of the skin**, bathe, and then apply dried and powdered plant, and then wrap. **For menstrual cramps**, boil an entire plant in 1-gallon water for 20 minutes. Drink three glasses per day. **For bee stings or other skin irritation**, crush the leaves and apply the juice.

China Root

Also known as wild sarsa, this deciduous vine has small, greenish flowers and a berry that is reddish-brown when ripe. It grows up into the forest canopy, and has a red, underground tuber. It is a relative of sarsasparilla, another medicinal herb.

WHERE IT CAN BE FOUND:

Tropical areas around the world

PROPERTIES AND USE:

Carminative, tonic, diuretic, digestive, detoxifier, febrifuge, hepatoprotective, antibiotic, diaphoretic, alterative, and treats exhaustion, anemia, acidity, toxicity, rheumatism, gout, lymphatic infection, skin conditions, male impotency

TRADITIONAL PREPARATION:

As a blood tonic, and for exhaustion, anemia, acidity, toxicity, rheumatism, gout, lymphatic infections, and skin conditions, boil a small handful of chopped roots in 3 cups water. **For impotency in men** with good prostate health (China root can stimulate prostate swelling), a handful of roots is soaked in rum and taken as a shot twice per day. Alternatively, boil 1 tablespoon China root powder in 1-quart water for 10 minutes. Remove from heat and steep for 10 minutes. Strain, and sip throughout the day. Repeat for three days, or until normal sexual function resumes. In the Caribbean, China root is soaked with man strength (Stemodia maritime L.) in rum for virility.

Chipilín

This shrub grows to 5 feet tall and has bright-yellow flowers clustered at the tips of the stems, usually with thorns. It is important as a foodstuff, as the leaves are rich in calcium, iron, thiamine, riboflavin, niacin, and ascorbic acid. Chipilín gives tamale dough its color and characteristic flavor. It is also used in traditional corn soup recipes in Honduras. Despite its popularity south of the border, Chipilín is considered a noxious weed in Hawaii.

WHERE IT CAN BE FOUND:

Mexico, Central America, Hawaii

PROPERTIES AND USE:

Nervine, suppurative. Used to treat anemia, pus-filled sores. Seeds and roots are toxic.

TRADITIONAL PREPARATION:

For nerves, 1 tablespoon leaves steeped in 1 cup boiling water. Cover, and let stand for 5 to 8 minutes. Strain and drink with honey.

Ciguapate

From the Náhautl words for "woman" and "medicine", ciguapate is a densely branched shrub with yellow flowers. It grows in temperate zones and reaches a height of 10 feet tall. Contrary to its name, it is beneficial to both sexes.

WHERE IT CAN BE FOUND:

Mexico, Central America

PROPERTIES AND USE:

Aphrodisiac, analgesic, diuretic, and used to treat headache, difficult labor, menstrual cramps, colic, and digestion problems

TRADITIONAL PREPARATION:

For all conditions, steep a small handful of the flowers in a liter of boiling water. Drink throughout the day. **For headaches**, place the leaves directly on the forehead.

Cinco Negritos

This shrub grows to between 3 and 10 feet in height. It has yellow to orange flowers that grow in dense heads and change to red or purple as they mature. The fruit grows in a drupe that turns black when ripened. Speaking to its medicinal powers, it is known in many lands by many names: wild sage, red sage, white sage, big sage, five little indians, cat's claw, *confiturio*, and *tickberry*. Great care must be taken when ingesting this herb, as it can be toxic.

WHERE IT CAN BE FOUND:

Mexico, Caribbean, Southern US, Central and South America, Asia-Pacific Region, Australia, New Zealand, Africa, Hawaii

PROPERTIES AND USE:

Antibacterial, antivenomous, antitumor, diuretic, tonic, febrifuge, hypotensive, carminative, antispasmodic, anti-inflammatory, antimalarial, antibacterial, insecticidal, antifungal, diaphoretic, hypoglycemic. Used to treat dysentery, diarrhea, vomiting, stomach pain, liver pain, toothache, epilepsy, cramps rashes, ulcers, insect bites, earache, deafness, pulmonary emphysema, cystic fibrosis, hepatitis, rheumatism, cough, flu, asthma, nausea, emotional stress.

TRADITIONAL PREPARATION:

Flowers are used in a tonic for rheumatism. **For earaches and to alleviate deafness**, place a large handful of flowers, chopped stems, and macerated leaves in coconut oil. Heat until the flowers wilt, and then remove from heat and allow to cool completely. Strain, and then pour into the affected ear(s). **To relieve itching or inflammation**, burn the leaves, and then grind into a powder. Apply directly to the affected area. Also, for itching and inflammation, place 9 leaves in a cool bath. **For all other conditions**, boil 1 large handful of the stems and root in 1-gallon water for 30 minutes. Allow too steep for 30 minutes. Strain, and drink three glasses per day.

Clavel

Derived from the Greek word meaning "flower of the gods", clavel, or carnation, has medicinal and spiritual powers revered since ancient times. This perennial herb grows to 4 feet high and has very narrow leaves and multi-petaled flowers with a light fragrance. The original flower color was a bright pinkish purple, but today, they are cultivated in many other shades.

WHERE IT CAN BE FOUND:

Mediterranean, Mexico, Central America, Arkansas, Massachusetts

PROPERTIES AND USE:

Nervine, antispasmodic, anti-inflammatory, tonic, diaphoretic, hypotensive, and used to treat heart disease, nausea, motion sickness, menopause symptoms, skin conditions, tired eyes, poor metabolism, Parkinson's disease, headache, anxiety, chest congestion, fatigue

TRADITIONAL PREPARATION:

For heart health, steep 1 teaspoon dried flowers per cup boiling water. Steep for 2 to 4 minutes. **For rashes and itching**, place flower heads in a cool bath. Can be used as a face wash to treat wrinkles, rosacea, and eczema.

AYURVEDIC CHEST CONGESTION AND FATIGUE CURE

Makes about 1 cup

This treatment comes to us from Ayurveda, the 5,000-year-old traditional Hindu medicine system.

INGREDIENTS:

- 1 cup water

- 1 cup sugar

- 1 tablespoon fresh carnation petals

INSTRUCTIONS:

- Bring to a boil, stirring until the sugar is completely dissolved.

USE:

- Allow to cool and drink a tablespoon per hour for three hours.

Coconut

This erect palm with an erect or slightly curved stem grows from a swollen base. The crown is made of 60 to 70 spirally arranged leaves comprised of 200 to 250 pinnately divided, tapering leaflets. Fruit is a single seed protected by a thick, stony shell partially filled with liquid. It can reach a height of 98 feet tall and live up to 90 years.

WHERE IT CAN BE FOUND:

Mexico, Central America, and tropical South America, Asia, Africa, Pacific region

PROPERTIES AND USE:

Anti-aging, antibacterial, antiviral, antifungal, febrifuge, antitumor, vermifuge. Treats abscesses, asthma, hair loss, colds, constipation, flu, skin conditions, sore throat, toothache, damaged hair, herpes, hepatitis, lice, candida, athletes' foot, thrush, diaper rash, SARS, AIDS.

TRADITIONAL PREPARATION:

To treat hair loss and damage, combine 1 tablespoon coconut oil and 1 tablespoon honey. Coat your hair and/or scalp and allow to sit for 40 minutes to 1 hour. For dry hair, rub just the ends. This same mixture treats skin conditions. **For acne,** wash the affected area with coconut water. **For sore throat,**

swallow 1 tablespoon warmed coconut oil. **To treat head lice**, rinse hair in apple cider vinegar, and allow to air dry. Smooth coconut oil through the strands and let sit 24 hours (sleeping with a shower cap). To treat cold sores, rub coconut oil on the affected area. **For weight loss**, consume 1 tablespoon coconut oil before breakfast. **To treat cancer**, you will need three young, small coconuts. Use a sharp knife to chip away the "dry skin" that lies under the shell and over the soft meat. Combine the chips with 1 cup aloe juice. Boil for 20 minutes. Strain, and sip throughout the day.

Coffee

This small tree grows to 18 feet in height, and has dark green, shiny leaves that are 2.5 to 8 inches in length. Its fragrant flowers are white, in clusters of two to nine. Its egg-shaped fruits grow to less than one-half inch long, and are green when young, and then turn red, and eventually blue-black.

WHERE IT CAN BE FOUND:

Indigenous to Ethiopia, now cultivated in tropical regions worldwide

PROPERTIES AND USE:

Nervine, stimulant, antidepressant, antivenomous, diuretic, infant febrifuge, contraceptive, hypertensive, and treats heart disease, headache, cancer (particularly lung, breast, and prostate), strokes, asthma, diabetes, skin conditions, gout, dandruff, wounds, obesity, diabetes

TRADITIONAL PREPARATION:

As a stimulant and as a diuretic, boil 3 coffee leaves in 1 cup water for 10 minutes. **For infant fever**, mash the shells of green, unroasted seeds and create a poultice that is applied directly on the head. According to Rosita Arvigo, **a long-lasting contraceptive** that lasts up to 1 year is prepared by boiling a handful of freshly picked green coffee beans in 3 cups water for 10 minutes. Drink throughout the day for three consecutive days.

KATIA'S COFFEE RUB
Makes 1 treatment

This novel use for used coffee grounds is great for relieving water retention, improving circulation, and diminishing the appearance of cellulite.

INGREDIENTS:

- 1/2 cup used coffee grounds

- 2 tablespoons oatmeal (optional)

- 3 tablespoon honey

- 1 tablespoon bergamot oil

INSTRUCTIONS:

- Mix well to combine and apply to the skin.

- Do not apply to the face and rinse off within 15 minutes.

USE:

Spread on by hand, or with a stiff-bristled brush. Do not apply to the face. Rinse off within 15 minutes.

DID YOU KNOW?

A recent study shows that coffee may protect men, but not women, against Parkinson's disease.

Contribo

A hairy vine that grows to 10 feet, with a strong and somewhat offensive odor. The leaves are dark green with three lobes, and a flower that when closed is pale pink, and when open, is speckled with brown and mauve. It is often described as having a heart or duck shape. It's also known as duck flower, Alcatraz, and *hierba del indio*.

WHERE IT CAN BE FOUND:

Mexico, Central America, South America, Caribbean

PROPERTIES AND USE:

Hypotensive, emmenagogue, antiparasitic, abortifacient, antivenomous. Treats hangovers, flu, colds, constipation, stomachache, indigestion, gas, gastritis, sinusitis, muscle pain.

TRADITIONAL PREPARATION:

For muscle pain, use an elastic bandage to apply the leaves directly to the affected area overnight. **For sinusitis**, soak a 6-inch piece of vine in 1-quart water in the sun all day. Sip over a 12-hour period. You can repeat this for a second day, if necessary. **For snakebites**, chew the leaves, and pack into the fang marks. **For all other ailments**, boil a handful of chopped vines in 3 cups water for 10 minutes. Strain, and drink warm before meals.

DID YOU KNOW?

Contribo soaked in rum, either alone or with other herbs such as China root (*Smilax* sp.) and man strength (*Stemodia maritime* L.), is so popular in the Caribbean and throughout most of Central America that it can be ordered in most taverns.

Copal

This papery-barked tree grows to 100 feet tall and has curved branches resembling an elephant trunk, giving copal its common name, elephant tree. It has large leathery leaves and has been used medicinally and ceremoniously by Mesoamerican people since pre-Columbian times.

WHERE IT CAN BE FOUND:

Mexico, Central America, Baja California, southwestern Arizona

PROPERTIES AND USE:

Antifungal, antiparasitic, febrifuge. Treats upper respiratory tract infections, and skin conditions such as scabies, funguses, dermatitis, impetigo. Also used to treat rheumatism, arthritis, insect bites, rashes, sore muscles, wounds, sores, dysentery, and dental cavities. Also used to ward off evil eye, black magic, and malicious spirits.

TRADITIONAL PREPARATION:

For toothache, stick a piece of the resin in the affected tooth. **For skin conditions**, scrape and powder the bark, and apply to the affected area. **For all conditions**, boil a 1-inch by 3-inch piece of bark. Boil in 1 cup water for 10 minutes. Drink before eating a meal. **For diarrhea**, add a 1-inch by 1-inch piece of copal to 1 cup water. Allow to sit overnight before drinking. **For fever**, make a cold infusion by mashing 3 leaves in 1-quart water, and soaking it overnight. Sip throughout the day.

Cordyceps

Introduced to the US in the mid-19th century, Cordyceps is farmed at high altitudes for medicinal use. Although not actually a mushroom, but rather a rare combination of a caterpillar and a parasitic fungus, it is often described as a medicinal mushroom. The base of the fungus first originates in an insect larval host (*Hepialus armoricanus*) and ends at a club-like cap. The fruit body is brown to black. When mature, the fungus consumes more than 90% of the infected insect and mummifies the host. Cordyceps contains all amino acids, and vitamins E, K, and B. It is used by professional athletes the world over.

WHERE IT CAN BE FOUND:

Tibet, China, Hawaii

PROPERTIES AND USE:

Anti-aging, aphrodisiac, adaptogen, tonic, anti-inflammatory, and treats diabetes, hepatitis, kidney disease, cancer, heart disease, cough, colds, bronchitis, male impotence, insomnia, anemia, fatigue, muscle pain, anemia, kidney disorders, dizziness, high cholesterol, heart arrhythmias, Lyme disease

TRADITIONAL PREPARATION:

For all ailments, add 1 teaspoon cordyceps sinensis powder to 1 cup hot water, hot chocolate, or coffee.

DID YOU KNOW?

Cordyceps sinesis is an effective tool for improving immune system function and the quality of life following chemotherapy.

Corn

The plant most revered by the Maya, corn is an annual, cultivated plant growing to 6.5 feet tall. Its leaves droop, and its seeds, known as kernels, grow on a woody axis known as an "ear". The color and size of the seeds vary greatly by region. It was originally domesticated in ancient times by the people of Mesoamerica.

WHERE IT CAN BE FOUND:

Midwest of the United States, as well as minor crop distribution elsewhere, predominantly on the East Coast; China; Mexico; Indonesia; India; France; Ukraine; South Africa; Brazil; Argentina; and minor distribution elsewhere

PROPERTIES AND USE:

Anti-inflammatory, astringent, diuretic. Treats ailments of the urinary tract, such as bladder infections and kidney troubles. Also used for hangovers, prostate health, liver ailments, lymphatic infections, bruising, skin conditions, arthritis, gout, bedwetting, gonorrhea, diarrhea.

TRADITIONAL PREPARATION:

For bruises, swelling, boils, and itching, mash uncooked corn kernels, and apply directly to the affected area for 1 hour. **For arthritis, gout, and water retention**, drink the cooled water in which fresh corn ears were boiled. **For bedwetting**, consume a cup before bedtime. **For diarrhea**, roast three cobs of corn. Remove the kernels, and grind into a paste. Stir into 1 cup room-temperature water, and drink in one sitting. **For gonorrhea and burning during urination**, boil a handful of corn, a pinch of gum arabic, and 2 tablespoons sugar with 3 cups water. Strain and sip throughout the day. **For all other ailments**, boil the silk from 3 ears of corn in 3 cups water for 5 minutes. Sip throughout the day.

CORN SILK TINCTURE
Makes 2 cups

This gentle yet effective tincture treats all listed conditions, and is especially great for bladder and kidney infections, water retention, and bedwetting. You will need a 16-ounce jar with lid for this recipe.

INGREDIENTS:

- 1/2 cup fresh, chopped corn silk

- 2 cups 100-proof vodka

INSTRUCTIONS:

- Pack a jar one-quarter full of fresh, chopped corn silk.

- Pour in 100-proof vodka to fill the jar.

- Tightly screw on the lid, and store in a cool, dark place for six weeks, shaking occasionally.

- Strain before use. The tincture should keep for up to 1 year.

USE:

- Take 1 teaspoon three times per day.

Cowfoot Vine

This woody, climbing vine grows to 20 inches long, with leaves in the shape of a cow's hoof and bright yellow flowers. In Central America, it can be found in forests and alongside the road.

WHERE IT CAN BE FOUND:

Yucatán Peninsula, Central America, Northwest South America

PROPERTIES AND USE:

Astringent, antihemorrhagic, and used to treat dysentery, headache, and internal wounds

TRADITIONAL PREPARATION:

For hemorrhaging, boil a 1-inch by 9-inch section of vine in 1-quart water for 10 minutes. Allow to cool. Drink throughout the day. **For internal bleeding**, drink sip two glasses of the same decoction in a 30-minute timeframe. **For headaches**, mash the leaves, and apply directly to the head. In the Maya lands, it is still in some parts used as a natural birth control, as it was in ancient times. According to Rosita Arvigo, one handful of the vine is boiled in 3 cups water for 10 minutes. A cup of this tea is consumed before each meal during menstruation. It is said that this dose is effective for up to six months. Drinking it during nine menstrual cycles will result in irreversible infertility.

Coyol Palm

This palm tree is spiny throughout, with pinnate leaves and edible fruits. Throughout Mexico, Central, and South America, the coyol palm's sap, flowers, fruits, and buds (called its "heart")

are used for medicine. In ancient times, it was revered by people throughout Mesoamerica, particularly at the Maya site of Copán. Numerous pottery vases, incense burners, and other pieces of art depicted the coyol palm, and plant remains were found in important tombs and throughout the Copán Valley. The earliest known medicinal use of coyol palm was in Mexico's Tehuacan Valley in 4,800 BC.

WHERE IT CAN BE FOUND:

Mexico, Central America, tropical South America

PROPERTIES AND USE:

Coyol palm fruit—the meat of which is similar to that of the coconut—has a high fat content, making it an important foodstuff, especially in times of scarcity and in impoverished regions. Anti-inflammatory, hypoglycemic. Remedy for bloody urine and diabetes. The flowers are used to brighten the mood. Sap, consumed fresh, is used as a diuretic.

TRADITIONAL PREPARATION:

For all conditions, place 1 tablespoon dried coyol root powder in 2 cups boiling water. Sip throughout the day.

Cuturro

This slender shrub has many branches and grows to 10 feet tall. Its branches and leaves are shiny, and its flowers are white or light green with spikes up to 3 inches long. It is widely available in Guatemala and Honduras, where it can be found growing in forests, in old fields, and on roadsides.

WHERE IT CAN BE FOUND:

Mexico, Central America

PROPERTIES AND USE:

Antivenomous, anti-inflammatory, sedative, emmenagogue, and used to treat skin conditions, fatigue, insomnia, toothache, headache, constipation, rheumatism, sore muscles, arthritis, cramping

TRADITIONAL PREPARATION:

For sore muscles, rheumatism, arthritis, cramping, and delayed menstruation or menstrual cramps, boil two large handfuls of fresh leaves in 1-gallon water for 15 to 20 minutes. Cool, and then use as a bath in which the person sits for at least 20 minutes. **For toothaches**, mash a bit of the root and place on or in the tooth. **For snakebites**, boil for 10 minutes in 3 cups water a piece of the root equal to the victim's arm. Administer while transporting to a hospital or healer. **For**

headache, constipation, and as a sedative, macerate the leaves and drink.

Cypress

Cupressus lusitanica grows in Mexico and Central America, and is the species used by the medicine men and women we have encountered. It is an evergreen that grows to at least 100 feet and has scale-like leaves. There are many species of cypress growing throughout the Northern Hemisphere. Unlike other herbs, which vary by species in their applications, all types of cypress have much the same use.

WHERE IT CAN BE FOUND:

Mexico and Central America

PROPERTIES AND USE:

Astringent, anti-aging, antiperspirant, antibacterial, antispasmodic, nervine, skin tonic, muscle relaxant, aromatic. Treats dandruff, bacterial or fungal skin infections, cellulite, varicose veins, broken capillaries, poor circulation, ovarian dysfunction. Wood used for incense. Foliage used for respiratory tract.

TRADITIONAL PREPARATION:

For dandruff, infuse 1 cup olive oil with a macerated 3-inch piece of foliage for 1 week. After 1 week, dilute with water, and use a small amount as a leave-in treatment on clean, towel-dried hair. You may wish to combine this with clary sage for aroma. This same oil is used as a massage oil **for cellulite, varicose veins, and poor circulation**. You may also use 10 drops cypress extract into sweet almond oil for this. **To calm the nerves**, boil a large handful of foliage in a quart of water. Slowly and deeply inhale the scent. Also, to calm the nerves, you may use a few drops of cypress oil in a warm bath. It's wonderful combined with rose, jasmine, or geranium oils.

DID YOU KNOW?

In Central America, cypress wood is used for incense in sacred ceremonies.

Dandelion

Taraxacum officinale is a plant from 2 to 6 inches or more with single yellow or orange rosette growing from a central taproot. The flowers are open during the day and closed at night. When broken, the stem exudes a white, milky latex. Mature heads turn white and disperse in the wind. It is high in vitamins A, B, C, and D, and in minerals such as iron, potassium, and zinc.

Dandelion found in the Caribbean, *Senna occidentalis*, aka piss-a-bed, wild coffee, and stinking weed, is used in the same manner.

WHERE IT CAN BE FOUND:

Throughout Europe, Asia, India, New Zealand, Australia, Southern Africa, the Americas

PROPERTIES AND USE:

Diuretic, laxative, hypotensive, digestive, blood tonic, alterative, anti-inflammatory. Used to treat warts, anorexia, gall bladder and liver issues, nausea, poor lactation, diabetes, eye infection, heartburn, kidney infection, diarrhea.

TRADITIONAL PREPARATION:

To make an infusion, pour 3 cups boiling water over 8 fresh dandelion heads or 2 tablespoons dried. Steep for 5 minutes. Sip throughout the day. **For a liver tonic and to treat systemic inflammation**, make dandelion "coffee" by roasting over low heat 4 tablespoons minced taproots that have been freshly harvested. When they begin to smell nutty, remove from heat. The longer you roast the roots, the stronger your coffee" will be. You may also perform this step by placing them on a baking sheet and baking for three hours at 150 degrees F. Use the roasted roots as you would coffee.

DANDELION TONIC
Makes about 2 cups

You will need a juicer for this recipe, which is excellent for cleansing.

INGREDIENTS:

- 3 cups dandelion root

- 10 carrots

- 6 Granny Smith apples

INSTRUCTIONS:

- Juice the items, and then stir well to combine.

- Chill for 1 hour, and then stir again before serving.

USE:

- Drink room temperature or chilled. To treat colds, flu, and congestion, add 1 clove garlic or 1/2 teaspoon cayenne pepper. Sip throughout the day.

DID YOU KNOW?

Like the flowers themselves, dandelion greens are excellent in salads. They're also wonderful added to soups, sandwiches, green juices, and are great sautéed. Make certain the dandelions you're using are not from yards treated with chemicals. To sauté

5 cups greens (Sounds like a lot, but they'll wilt!), heat 2 tablespoons sesame oil in a large sauté pan over medium-high heat. Add the greens and sauté for 20 to 30 seconds. Season to taste with salt and freshly ground black pepper. Garnish with toasted sesame seeds. Dandelion greens are also delicious sautéed simply in a bit of olive oil.

Dead and Wake Prickle

This creeping annual or perennial herb goes by several common names, including twelve o'clock, prickle, *dormilón*, touch-me-not, shameplant, sleeping grass, and prayer plant. It has pinnate leaves that fold up when touched, and fluffy flowers that are lilac in color. It spreads up to 2 feet and grows in the shade.

WHERE IT CAN BE FOUND:

Central America, South America, Caribbean, East Africa, Australia

PROPERTIES AND USE:

Purgative, emetic, antibacterial, antifungal, hemorrhagic, antivenomous, sedative, antidepressant, antispasmodic, analgesic, hypotensive, nervine. Treats anxiety; inflammation; insomnia; skin conditions; urinary tract issues; diarrhea, dysentery, and other gastrointestinal problems; sinusitis;

lymphatic infections; asthma and other respiratory conditions; vaginal discomfort; fatigue; diabetes; toothache; arthritis; rheumatism; hemorrhoids; obesity; backache; kidney stones; bruises.

TRADITIONAL PREPARATION:

For insomnia, place it on the pillow before sleep. As an antispasmodic, diuretic, relaxant, pain reliever, and sleep inducer, boil 9 branches with leaves in 3 cups water for 5 minutes. Drink 1/2 cup three to six times daily as needed. **For diabetes or obesity**, boil a large handful of leaves in 1-gallon water for 30 minutes. Drink throughout the day. **To calm babies or induce sleep**, place a 1-inch piece of leaf in a bottle milk. It is typical in the Caribbean, and elsewhere in Central America, to place bunches of leaves in a cross formation in a baby's bed. Four crosses are used for babies and children (placed under the pillow), and nine for adults. **For kidney stones**, boil a handful of chopped roots in 1-gallon water for 30 minutes. Take three times per day before meals. **For kidney pain**, warm a few leaves, and apply them directly to the affected area. **For muscle spasms, backache, and nervous irritability or anxiety**, dry leaves in an oven set to 100 degrees F until the leaves are dried; the amount of time will vary on humidity levels and altitude. Remove the leaves from their stems, and powder lightly. Smoke as you would tobacco. For bruises, apply the bruised leaves to the affected area. **For**

toothache, gargle with the above infusion, or boil and mash the root as a poultice.

Echinacea

Echinacea is an herbaceous plant with spindle-shaped taproots that are usually branched. It grows up to 28 inches tall and has hairy stems and leaves. The petals are light purple to pink in color. It has for centuries been used as medicine by Native Americans.

WHERE IT CAN BE FOUND:

Colorado, Iowa, Kansas, Louisiana, Minnesota, Montana, Missouri, North Dakota, Nebraska, Oklahoma, South Dakota, Texas, Wyoming, Manitoba, Saskatchewan

PROPERTIES AND USE:

Anti-inflammatory, antibacterial, antiviral, antivenomous, emetic, antimalarial, and treats candida, colds, earache, immune deficiency, insect bites, sinusitis, sore throat, herpes, streptococcus infections, migraines, chronic fatigue syndrome, ADHD, hemorrhoids, syphilis

TRADITIONAL PREPARATION:

For all conditions, use Echinacea Tincture as described. To make an infusion, add a small handful of Echinacea root to 1-

liter water and bring to a boil. Boil, covered, for 10 minutes. Remove from heat and allow too steep for 30 minutes. Strain, and sip throughout the day. For yeast infections, melt 1/2 cup chopped beeswax in a double boiler. Stir in 1 cup dried Echinacea and 1 cup olive oil. Remove from heat. Stir in the contents of 2 vitamin E capsules. When cooled, place in a jar with lid. Apply directly to the affected area. You may also make it into a vaginal suppository.

ECHINACEA TINCTURE
Makes 1 quart

This tincture is especially effective for proper immune system function. You will need a quart sized jar with lid for this recipe.

INGREDIENTS:

- 1 cup finely chopped Echinacea root

- 1-quart 100-proof vodka

INSTRUCTIONS:

- Place the Echinacea root in the jar.

- Pour in 100-proof vodka to fill the jar.

- Tightly screw on the lid, and place on a windowsill too steep for six weeks.

- The tincture should keep for up to 3 years.

USE:

Take 1/2 teaspoon every 2 hours for acute conditions, or three times per day for chronic conditions.

Epazote

Epazote is an aromatic herb growing to 40 inches, with small ovate or lanceolate, sharply toothed leaves that are green in color. It is high in minerals, but not vitamins. It does, however, contain vitamins A and B, as well as beta-carotenes. It is an excellent source of folic acid. It is also known as *ipazote*, *pazote*, quinoa, *epasote*, goosefoot, wormseed, and Mexican tea.

WHERE IT CAN BE FOUND:

Central America, Mexico, Caribbean, most of the US and Canada, tropical and subtropical regions worldwide

PROPERTIES AND USE:

Antifungal, vermifuge, anti-inflammatory, diaphoretic, febrifuge, abortifacient, sedative, anti-flatulent. Used for delayed menstruation, menstrual cramps, chills, dysentery, indigestion, gas, hangovers, asthma, dysentery, joint pain, respiratory problems, difficult childbirth. In addition to these conditions, Dysphania ambrosioides' more pungent cousin, epazote del zorrillo (Chenopodium graveolens), is used to treat depression, vomiting, and urinary conditions. Both can be toxic to animals.

TRADITIONAL PREPARATION:

For hangovers, boil an entire plant (excluding the roots) in 1-quart water with a dash of salt. Drink warm every 30 minutes until symptoms dissipate. **As a vermifuge**, take 1 teaspoon of the juice of mashed leaves alone, or added to milk, upon waking. As a sedative, boil 3 small branches in 2 cups water for 10 minutes. Drink while hot. **For athlete's foot**, place the leaves as a poultice directly on the affected area. For those prone to flatulence, add 1 to 2 sprigs per dish. It goes well with beans, mushrooms, corn, fish, chicken, and seafood.

DID YOU KNOW?

Epazote is a cousin of quinoa (C. quinoa).

Eucalyptus

This fast-growing, flowering evergreen tree can reach 200 feet tall. Its leaves are leathery, and its flowers in bud state are covered in a cup-like membrane (from where it gets its name, from the Greek *eucalyptos*, meaning "well covered"). This membrane falls off when the flower expands.

WHERE IT CAN BE FOUND:

Australia, Mediterranean, South America, parts of Central America

PROPERTIES AND USE:

Antispasmodic, rubefacient, antiviral, antibacterial, antifungal, anti-aging, anti-inflammatory, antiseptic, expectorant, insecticidal. Not only a sinus decongestant, but in parts of Mexico and Central America, a tea made of Eucalyptus leaves is used to decongest the liver, bladder, and kidneys. Treats gastritis, diabetes, liver disease, colds, flu, sore throat, bronchitis, catarrh, epilepsy, rheumatism, herpes, candida, migraine, ulcers, wounds, eye infection, asthma, acne, rheumatism, minor burns.

TRADITIONAL PREPARATION:

To make a basic tea, pour 1 cup boiling water over 1/2 teaspoon dried Eucalyptus leaves. Cover, and allow too steep for 10 minutes. Strain. You may wish to serve sweetened with honey or stevia. **For asthma, bronchitis, and other respiratory conditions**, add 1/2 teaspoon dried coltsfoot leaves and 1-ounce dried thyme leaves to the basic tea recipe. **For head colds**, add 2 teaspoons dried peppermint leaves and 1 teaspoon dried chamomile flowers to the basic tea recipe. **For sinus congestion**, place a towel over the head, and inhale the steam from the Eucalyptus tea. **For rheumatism and minor burns**, soak a clean cotton cloth in the cooled basic tea, and apply directly to the affected area two to three times per day. **For sore throats**, make a gargle with equal parts dried eucalyptus and dried calendula flowers. Gargle three times per day as needed.

DID YOU KNOW?

The tissue-constricting tannins in Eucalyptus make it an effective remedy for bleeding gums. Simply rinse with the cooled basic tea recipe twice per day.

Feverfew

A member of the daisy family, feverfew has citrus-scented leaves and grows to 18 inches tall. Though it is effective in treating allergies, it is not recommended for those who are allergic to other members of the daisy family, including ragweed and chrysanthemums. It is also not recommended for pregnant women, as it may cause the uterus to contract. Feverfew is also known as bachelor's buttons and featherfew.

WHERE IT CAN BE FOUND:

Eastern Europe, Mexico, Central America, South America, British Columbia, Manitoba, Ontario, Quebec, parts of Newfoundland and Labrador, and all US states except North Dakota, South Dakota, Iowa, Nebraska, Kansas, Oklahoma,

Texas, Arkansas, Louisiana, Georgia, Florida, Tennessee, Virginia, Arizona, New Mexico

PROPERTIES AND USE:

Anti-inflammatory, antispasmodic, emmenagogue, antitumor, anti-allergen, and used to treat painful menstruation, difficult childbirth, asthma, dizziness, tinnitus, nausea, vomiting, migraine, rheumatoid arthritis, psoriasis, insect bites, infertility, toothache

TRADITIONAL PREPARATION:

Eating the leaves is advised for all conditions. They're lovely in salads. To make an infusion, pour 1 cup boiling water over 1 teaspoon dried leaves. Steep for 5 to 8 minutes, and then strain. You may also use the flowers and stems in an infusion. **For insect bites**, rub the flower head on the affected area. **For toothache**, use the infusion as a gargle, or chew the flowers and stems.

Flax

Grown in cooler regions the world over, flax, also known as linseed, is an upright food and fiber plant growing to 4 feet tall. Its flowers are pale blue, and its fruit, a round, dry capsule, contains several small, brown seeds. Its Latin name, *Linum usitatissimum*, means "most useful". It is packed with omega-3 fatty acids.

WHERE IT CAN BE FOUND:

Eastern Mediterranean; Western Asia; the Middle East; Mexico; Central America; the entire US, except Nevada, Alaska, Hawaii, and New Mexico; all of Canada, except Yukon, Newfoundland, and Nunavut

PROPERTIES AND USE:

Astringent, hypotensive, nervine. Used to treat burns, cancer, constipation, poor vision, dry eyes, lupus, rheumatoid arthritis, osteoarthritis, ulcers, gastritis, heart disease, poor digestion, ADHD, obesity, dry skin, vaginal infections, benign prostatic hyperplasia, menopausal symptoms, high cholesterol, poor kidney function. It is said to prevent breast and prostate cancer.

TRADITIONAL PREPARATION:

For dry skin, take 1 teaspoon flaxseed oil before breakfast. You may also rub it directly onto the skin. **For high cholesterol**, consume 40 to 50 grams of flaxseed per day. Baked goods containing ground flaxseed are a good way to meet this requirement. **For kidney issues or lupus**, consume 15 grams of ground flaxseed twice daily. Cereal is a good way to consume this amount. **For menopausal symptoms**, consume 40 grams of crushed flaxseed per day.

Florifudia

When traveling in Guatemala, a local remarked about florifundia, "It's like a beautiful woman. It lures you in, and though one taste can be sweet, more can be deadly." Indeed, florifundia—also known as angel's trumpet—is a hallucinogen that can be extremely dangerous in high doses. Also known as toé in the Amazon, only the most experienced shamans may administer it. It is an evergreen shrub that reaches 23 feet in height. The leaves, flower stalks, fruit, and young shoots are covered in a velvety, white down. The five -pointed flowers are strongly fragrant at night, are trumpet-shaped, and point down. In bud state, they are yellow. Upon first opening, they are white. They are pink in maturity.

WHERE IT CAN BE FOUND:

Central America, South America, Spain, and India

PROPERTIES AND USE:

Febrifuge, antiparasitic, analgesic, antitumor, anti-inflammatory, decongestant. Used for arthritis, ulcers, backache, sore muscles, rheumatism, skin diseases, sciatica, dandruff, insomnia.

TRADITIONAL PREPARATION:

For insomnia, place a flower under or on top of your pillow. **For backaches, sore muscles, and rheumatism**, make a poultice with the leaves, and apply directly to the affected area. **For inflammation**, add 1 leaf to a cool bath.

DID YOU KNOW?

For centuries, this plant has been used in Mesoamerican shamanic rituals. It is used for divining, warding off evil spirits, and for black magic and sorcery. Combined with Cannabis indica and tobacco, its dry leaves are smoked. Crushed seeds are added to chichi, a psychoactive maize beer. In the Amazon jungle regions of Peru, the leaves are added to another psychoactive beverage that contains *Trichocereus pachanoi*.

Garlic

This bulbous plant has been used for medicinal purposes for thousands of years. Some consider it to be the most valuable herb yet discovered because of its multitude of culinary and medicinal applications. It grows to 4 feet in height, and is a relative of the onion, the shallot, the leek, the chive, and the rakkyo. Among its many properties, it keeps insects at bay, which is why it is included in most Spanish tapas. Interestingly, one of the most popular types of garlic sold in the US, so-called elephant garlic, is actually a wild leek (*Allium ampeloprasum*). This explains its much milder flavor profile.

WHERE IT CAN BE FOUND:

Mild climates worldwide

PROPERTIES AND USE:

Antibiotic, hypotensive, febrifuge, antitumor, hypoglycemic, antifungal, antibacterial. Treats vaginal infections, hay fever, diabetes, diarrhea, preeclampsia, colds, flu, rheumatism, gout, sinusitis, poor liver function, high cholesterol, earache, heart disease.

TRADITIONAL PREPARATION:

For sinusitis, boil 1 clove garlic in 1 cup water for 15 minutes. Allow to cool to room temperature, and then use as a nasal wash with a neti pot. **For vaginal infections**, place 1 or 2 whole, peeled cloves into the vagina at bedtime. In the morning, discard. Repeat for an additional night or two as needed. For serious infections, you may cut the clove in two; however, this might cause some mild stinging at first. **For earaches**, sauté one clove garlic in 1/4 cup olive oil. Allow to cool and pour the oil directly into the affected ear(s). You may instead soak the clove in the oil for a few days. Alternatively, you can insert a small clove directly into the affected ear(s). **For athlete's foot or ringworm**, steep an entire garlic bulb in 4 cups water. Soak the feet for 20 minutes, three times per day. For colds or flu, eat 3 fresh cloves at the onset of symptoms.

DID YOU KNOW?

According to the National Cancer Institute, preliminary studies suggest that eating garlic may reduce the risk of certain cancers, especially those on the gastrointestinal tract (stomach, colon, esophagus, pancreas).

Ginger

An herbaceous perennial reaching up to 3 feet tall in the wild, ginger grows from a fleshy, tuberous rhizome that is aromatic, thick-lobed, and pale yellowish. Its flowers are pale green to greenish-yellow with dark purple tips. Its health properties are revered the world over.

WHERE IT CAN BE FOUND:

North America, Central America, South America, and tropical Africa and Asia

PROPERTIES AND USE:

Stimulant, anti-flatulent, anti-inflammatory, hypotensive, febrifuge, carminative, tonic, and is used to treat gastritis, motion sickness, nausea, rheumatism, arthritis, sore muscles, colds, bronchitis, toothache, headache, cramps, difficult labor, poor lactation, high cholesterol, poor immune system function, earache. It is also used to prevent internal blood clots and heart disease.

TRADITIONAL PREPARATION:

For rheumatism and arthritis, slice fresh ginger and add to your meals. You may also add powdered ginger root to your food or beverages. **For gastritis, motion sickness, nausea, poor immune system function, poor lactation, and difficult labor**, cut a 2-inch piece of ginger into thin slices, and place in 1 cup water over low heat. Simmer, covered, for 10 minutes. Strain, and then sip in one sitting. For best results, consume 3 cups per day. **For chest colds, rheumatism, and sore muscles**, you may soak cotton or flannel cloth in the hot liquid and apply directly to the affected area. Repeat the treatment six times.

AYURVEDIC HEADACHE TREATMENT
Makes 1 treatment

This ancient treatment is simple and effective, giving prompt relief to even the most severe headache.

INGREDIENTS:

- One 2-inch piece of peeled ginger

INSTRUCTIONS:

- In a food processor, create a paste from the peeled ginger. You may also create a paste by mashing the ginger with the edge of a chef's knife

- Apply directly to the temples.

USE:

For added relief, inhale the vapor of 1 tablespoon dried ginger root powder in 1 cup boiling water. This vapor is excellent for colds, as well, and may be drunk after inhalation.

DID YOU KNOW?

If you're looking for a caffeine-free pick me up, grate a 1-inch piece of ginger in 1 cup warm water. Drink in one sitting.

Ginseng (American or Asian, not Siberian)

Ginseng is the root of plant in the genus Panax, such as Korean ginseng, South China ginseng and American ginseng.

WHERE IT CAN BE FOUND:

In the United States from the Midwest to Maine, primarily in the Appalachian and Ozark regions. It is also found in Eastern Canada, Manchuria in China, Japan and Korea.

PROPERTIES AND USE:

It can boost energy, reduce stress, aid in weight loss, and treat sexual issues such as loss of libido. It improves breathing, lowers blood sugar levels, supports the immune system, and reduces inflammation.

TRADITIONAL PREPARATION:

Ginseng can be used as a tea or taken in capsule form.

DID YOU KNOW?

Those with heart conditions, diabetes, or a manic mental disorder should avoid ginseng. It might also trigger bleeding. Those with hormonally-related cancers such as ovarian cancer should not use ginseng.

Goldenseal

A popular herbal supplement, goldenseal grows wild in some areas of the US, but has recently been listed as endangered because of overharvesting. Now goldenseal is grown commercially to provide for its demand. It gained its name from the golden coloring that shows up in the scars near the stem base. Historically, it was used by Native Americans for a number of health conditions, including ulcers, skin diseases, and gonorrhea. The stems of the plant are often dried for use in teas, and extracts are used in capsules and tablets. This supplement has gained popularity because of the reputation as an immune system booster and an herbal antibiotic.

WHERE IT CAN BE FOUND:

Alabama, Connecticut, Delaware, Georgia, Iowa, Illinois, Kansas, Kentucky, Massachusetts, Mississippi, Missouri, North Carolina, New Jersey, New York, Ohio, Oklahoma, Pennsylvania, Wisconsin, West Virginia, Canada, Blue Ridge Mountains and the deep wood mountain areas between Arkansas and Vermont

PROPERTIES AND USE:

Hypotensive, hypoglycemic, and antibiotic. It is used to treat colds, whooping cough, respiratory infections, stuffy nose, hay fever. It can also help with digestive problems, including infectious diarrhea, ulcers, stomach pain, intestinal gas, and constipation. It is also beneficial for skin conditions, such as rashes, herpes blisters, dandruff, cold sores, eczema, ringworm, and wounds. Fights cancer cells and treats vaginitis, eye infections, canker sores, gum irritation, gonorrhea, malaria, urinary tract infections, earache, and high cholesterol.

TRADITIONAL PREPARATION:

Goldenseal can be used topically as a wash or as a poultice **to cleanse wounds and treat various skin ailments**. **For oral ailments**, it can be mixed with water and used as a mouthwash. The fresh plant may cause mucous membrane inflammation, and so it might be best used as a dried herb, powder, or tincture. It is often combined with echinacea for maximum immune-boosting benefits. Because of the bitter taste, many people prefer to take it in a capsule.

DID YOU KNOW?

When a broken goldenseal stem heals, it looks like a golden wax seal on a letter. Hence, its name.

Guava

The guava tree grows to more than 30 feet tall. It has slender stems with dark brown bark that flakes, exposing a greenish layer beneath. The leaves are leathery, with white flowers at the ends of the branches. The fruit is rounded, 2.5 inches long, and turns yellow or pink when ripe. It is an excellent source of vitamin C. The fruit, leaves, and juice are used as medicine.

WHERE IT CAN BE FOUND:

Mexico, Central America, Northern South America, Caribbean, Africa, Southeast Asia, Mediterranean, Florida, Hawaii, Louisiana

PROPERTIES AND USE:

Hypotensive, antibacterial, antifungal, antiparasitic, analgesic, antispasmodic, heart tonic, hypoglycemic, emmenagogue, anti-aging, and used to treat candida, diarrhea, dysentery, nausea, dizziness, mouth sores, bleeding gums, halitosis, vomiting, cough, skin sores, wounds, conjunctivitis

TRADITIONAL PREPARATION:

To make an infusion, pour 3 cups boiling water over 1 cup guava leaves. Steep for 20 minutes. Drink, or use as a gargle **for mouth sores, bleeding gums, and halitosis**. **For diarrhea, nausea, dizziness, dysentery, and sore throats**, boil a 1-inch by 2-inch piece of bark in 3 cups water for 10 minutes. Take 1 cup before meals. Use as a rinse **for skin sores and wounds**. For conjunctivitis, macerate the leaves and apply as a poultice.

DID YOU KNOW?

According to Rosita Arvigo, in Belize, a remedy for diarrhea, dysentery, nausea, and colds is to boil 9 leaves and 9 young fruits in 3 cups water for 10 minutes. One cup of the warm decoction is drunk before meals.

Gumbo-limbo

Growing to more than 80 feet tall, the gumbo-limbo tree is known for its red, shaggy bark, which peels off in papery strips. It is this characteristic that gives it its common names—tourist tree and naked Indian—in Central America, where tourists suffering from red, peeling sunburn are a common sight.

WHERE IT CAN BE FOUND:

Mexico, Central America, tropical South America, Caribbean, Florida

PROPERTIES AND USE:

Febrifuge, anti-inflammatory, tonic, and treats skin conditions, sunburn, measles, internal infections, urinary tract infections, sun stroke, colds, flu, kidney infections, anemia, gout, headache

TRADITIONAL PREPARATION:

For skin conditions including blisters, swelling, exposure to poisonous plants, measles, sores, and itching, boil a 1-inch by 12-inch piece of bark in 1-gallon water for 10 minutes. Allow to cool completely, and then bathe the affected area three times daily. **For all other conditions except kidney infections,** consume this same preparation as a tea. **For kidney infections,** boil a 6-inch by 10-inch piece of bark in 3 quarts water for 10 minutes. Drink throughout the day in place of water. **For headache**, apply the leaves directly to the forehead.

Hawthorn

This hardy tree grows to 30 feet tall, and has pendulous branches with dark, shiny, serrated leaves. It has scaly bark that is reddish-brown in youth and grey when older. It grows dense, rose-like flowers that have a fi shy odor that attracts pollinators. Its red berries are used to make pies and preserves.

WHERE IT CAN BE FOUND:

Most of Canada, Alaska, Washington, Oregon, California, Nevada, Montana, Wyoming, North Dakota, South Dakota, Minnesota, Wisconsin, Michigan

PROPERTIES AND USE:

Diuretic, astringent, tonic, anti-inflammatory, and used to treat heart conditions, sore throat, kidney conditions, edema, diarrhea, dysentery, and STDs

TRADITIONAL PREPARATION:

For all conditions, boil 1 handful berries in 1-quart water for 30 minutes. Strain, and drink 1 cup per day.

Hibiscus

Known as *flor de Jamaica* by most we encountered in the Maya lands, Hibiscus is also called tulipán by Spanish-speaking peoples the world over. It is a woody shrub that grows to 26 feet tall. It has slender stems and many branches. The flowers are bright red and have yellow stamen tubes. Elsewhere, trumpet-shaped relatives in the Hibiscus family may be red, orange, purple, pink yellow, or white. These flowers do not have known medicinal properties. The red Hibiscus is the Hindu goddess Kali's flower. Like her, it symbolizes time and change, death and rebirth. In Hindu worship, it is offered to both Kali and to Lord Ganesha.

WHERE IT CAN BE FOUND:

Tropical and subtropical regions the world over, Southern Texas, Florida, Southern California, Hawaii

PROPERTIES AND USE:

Hypotensive, diuretic, expectorant, nervine, suppurative, and used to treat insomnia, poor circulation, constipation, high cholesterol, stomach conditions, colds, cough, nerve diseases, hair loss, heart weakness, cellulite, postpartum hemorrhages, excess menstrual flow, skin conditions, headache, painful menstruation, and to prevent miscarriages

TRADITIONAL PREPARATION:

For all conditions, bring 1 cup water just to a boil. Pour over 2 teaspoons dried hibiscus flowers. Steep for 5 minutes. **For hair loss and to keep hair lustrous**, sauté 2 tablespoons dried hibiscus flowers in 1/4 cup coconut oil for 2 minutes. Add 2 curry leaves, and 1 teaspoon gooseberry. Allow to cool, and then spread on the hair and scalp. You may also juice the leaves and apply to the hair and scalp for 45 minutes to 1 hour. The juice may also be used to treat cellulite.

DID YOU KNOW?

In Rosita Arvigo's fabulous book Rainforest Remedies: One Hundred Healing Herbs of Belize, she explains that a wife whose husband has strayed but still loves her may prepare Hibiscus tea to entice him to return to her. She explains that nine leaves and nine open flowers are boiled in 3 quarts water for 10 minutes. Each day for nine days, she gives her husband 1 cup of the decoction to drink and bathes him with the remainder.

Hierba Mora

This short-lived perennial herb has an erect, angular, branching stem that grows to 2 feet high and may be covered with inward-bent hair. The alternate leaves are dark green, ovate, and wavy toothed. Its fruit is a pea-sized, black or purple berry containing many seeds. Its flowers are white. It is also known as black nightshade.

WHERE IT CAN BE FOUND:

Europe, Western Asia, Australia, South Africa, Mexico, Central America, Caribbean, British Columbia, Alberta, Manitoba, Ontario, Quebec, Newfoundland, Alaska, Alabama, California, Connecticut, District of Columbia, Florida, Hawaii, Massachusetts, Maryland, Maine, New Hampshire, New Jersey, New York, Oregon, South Carolina, Virginia, Washington

PROPERTIES AND USE:

Nervine, sedative, antimalarial, anti-inflammatory, febrifuge, antifungal, stomachic, analgesic, and used to treat hepatitis, burns, skin conditions, vaginal infections, diabetes, rheumatism, liver disease, wounds, respiratory infections

TRADITIONAL PREPARATION:

For fever, boil 1 to 2 dried leaves in 1 cup water. Cool, and then drink in one sitting. **For inflammation, burns, and rheumatism**, bruise the fresh leaves, and apply directly to the skin. **For skin conditions and fungal infections**, macerate the leaves, and apply the juice directly to the affected area. **For skin conditions, as well as for wounds and vaginal infections**, boil, covered, a large handful of the stalk, leaves, and roots for 20 minutes. Allow to cool. Drink throughout the day. **For respiratory infections, acne flare ups, pain, and fevers**, juice the leaves and berries and drink 1/2 cup per day. As a stomachic, steep a small handful of the flower buds with 1 tablespoon salt in 1-liter water. This can also be used as a wash for wounds or skin conditions.

Holy Basil

A short-lived, aromatic perennial that grows to 3 feet tall, holy basil is erect, with fi ne hair and nearly round leaves. The flowers are purple or reddish. It is known as *tulsi* ("beyond compare") in India, where it is a sacred plant used widely in worship, cooking, and medicine.

WHERE IT CAN BE FOUND:

Caribbean, Central America, South America, South Asia, Malaysia

PROPERTIES AND USE:

Adaptogen, antibacterial, expectorant, analgesic, antifungal, nervine, carminative, tonic, hypotensive, antispasmodic, hypoglycemic, antiparasitic, anti-allergen, and is used to treat ulcers, viral infections, depression, respiratory infection, cough, colds, flu , herpes, poor immune system function, headache, indecision, dulled senses, and radiation exposure

TRADITIONAL PREPARATION:

For all conditions, boil 2 tablespoons dried holy basil in 8 ounces water for 10 minutes. Prepare twice per day, and drink while hot. **For all conditions**, you may also juice the leaves, setting your juicer to low. Take up to 2 tablespoons per day. **For fungal infections**, rub the leaves directly on the affected area. For athletes' foot, place the leaves in your socks overnight. To make a tincture, place 1 cup dried holy basil leaf in a glass, one-quart jar. Fill to the top with 100-proof, whole-grain alcohol. Store a cool, dark place, shaking daily, for six weeks. Drink 1 to 2 drops once or twice daily.

DID YOU KNOW?

In Hindu mythology, holy basil is the incarnation of the goddess of divine protection, Tulsi. In Ayurveda, it is used to reduce Kapha, or the amount of "earth" in your dosha, or mind-body type. If used in excess, it can have an aggravating effect on Pitta, or the fi re dosha. Because of this, it's good for someone who is suffering from a Kapha imbalance, and therefore feels "stuck in a rut".

HOLY BASIL OIL
Makes 1 cup

This oil is great brushed on chicken or vegetables, or combined with cilantro, parsley, and 1 dried ancho chili. It can be used to create a medicinal vinaigrette.

INGREDIENTS:

- 1 1/2 cups packed fresh holy basil leaves

- 3/4 cup extra virgin olive oil

INSTRUCTIONS:

- Bring a medium pot of water to a boil. Remove from heat and blanch the basil for 10 seconds.

- Drain, and rinse under cold, running water. Pat basil dry with plain, white paper towels.

- Place in a blender. Add the oil in a slow, steady stream. Blend until smooth. Season with sea salt and freshly ground white pepper.

- Allow to cool, and then cover and chill.

USE:

Use within three days.

Horsetail

The second-largest horsetail, this species grows to more than 16 feet tall. It has the thickest stem and bears many whorls of slender branches. Some of them terminate in spore cones. *Equisetum fluviatile* L., the horsetail species that grows in nearly all US states, and throughout Europe, Russia, Korea, New

Zealand, and Canada, has the same medicinal properties as the giant species we encountered in Central America. It is a prehistoric herb that can be dangerous in abnormally high doses.

WHERE IT CAN BE FOUND:

Central America, Mexico, central Chile to Brazil

PROPERTIES AND USE:

Diuretic, hypotensive, antifungal, anti-inflammatory, analgesic, febrifuge, antitumor, suppurative, antihemorrhagic, and used to treat hair loss, arthritis, osteoporosis, obesity, hepatitis, tuberculosis, jaundice, skin conditions, urinary tract infections, broken bones, muscle cramps, nosebleeds, brittle nails, respiratory infections, renal conditions, wounds

TRADITIONAL PREPARATION:

For muscle cramps, arthritis, and skin conditions, soak a handful of dried horsetails in 1-gallon lukewarm water for 15 minutes. Drip a cheesecloth in the water and place the soaked herb in the cloth. Apply it as a hot or cold compress on the affected area. Repeat two to three times per day. **To reduce inflammation and pain**, grind the plant into a paste, and apply directly to the affected area. This is especially successful when used after a compress. **For brittle nails**, steep 1 tablespoon dried horsetail in 1 cup boiling water for 10 minutes.

Allow to cool and soak the nails in the infusion for 20 minutes. After soaking, apply extra-virgin olive oil to soften the cuticles. This is best if done before bed and used in conjunction with gloves while you sleep. Repeat three times per week. This infusion is also effective in treating hair with split ends. **For all other conditions**, make an infusion by steeping a small handful of dried horsetails (or two large handfuls fresh) in 1-liter boiling water for 10 minutes. Sip throughout the day. When cooled, this same infusion can be used as a skin or hair rinse. For athlete's foot, mix 1 cup chopped, fresh horsetail with 4 cups boiling apple cider vinegar. Steep overnight. Use as a foot soak for 10 days. **For wounds**, boil, covered, a small handful of fresh horsetails for 20 minutes. Allow to cool, and then apply to the wounds. This is also effective in stopping bleeding.

Huito

Genipa americana is known by many names, including *danipa, genipayer bito, maluco,* and *jagua*. It is a medium-sized tropical tree that typically grows to 65 feet. It has smooth bark, a dense crown, and horizontal lower branches. Its fruit is a large berry that is used for medicine and to make beverages.

WHERE IT CAN BE FOUND:

Mexico, Caribbean, Central America, South America

PROPERTIES AND USE:

Abortifacient, cholagogue, diuretic, antiseptic, tonic, stomachic, laxative, antitumor, astringent, and used to treat respiratory conditions, vaginitis, catarrh, diarrhea, uterine cancer, skin ulcers, anemia, insect bites, gonorrhea, jaundice

TRADITIONAL PREPARATION:

Consume 1 cup per day of the berry, or drink 1 cup juice.

DID YOU KNOW?

When mature, the berry turns jet black. It is used by South American Indians as body paint.

Hyacinth

Known for its association with the Hyacinthus of Greek mythology, this plant has been used medicinally since ancient times. Though it was more widely used in the past, it is still used today. Hyacinth's bulb is a sturdy base that grows the stem, which blooms between the months of April and May bluebell flowers that are purple-bluish in color. It is also commonly known as the bluebell plant or wild hyacinth.

WHERE IT CAN BE FOUND:

Great Britain, Western Europe, the Pacific Northwest, Indiana, Kentucky, New Jersey, New York, Ohio, Pennsylvania, Virginia

PROPERTIES AND USE:

Diuretic, insecticide, and treats HIV and cancer

TRADITIONAL PREPARATION:

For all conditions, dry and powder the bulb. (Fresh bulbs are poisonous.) To make an infusion, stir 1 teaspoon dried bulb powder in 1 cup boiling water. Sip throughout the day.

DID YOU KNOW?

Legend holds that Apollo was grief-stricken over the death of his love, Hyacinthus, and as a result raised the purple flower we know as the hyacinth. For centuries, the flowers were used for grief and mourning. To this day, some carry a sprig of hyacinth near their hearts.

Inga

This tree grows to 55 feet tall, and has a broad, spreading crown that is nearly flat. The leaves are simply pinnate, with four to six pairs of large, oval leaflets. Its flowers are usually white, and its seeds are covered by a sweet, white powder. The pulp tastes like vanilla ice cream, hence its common name, ice cream bean. In Central America, Inga trees can be seen growing at coffee plantations, where they provide great shade. They attract hummingbirds and are therefore popular planted near windows.

WHERE IT CAN BE FOUND:

Mexico, Central America, Amazon forest region, Africa

PROPERTIES AND USE:

Used to treat wounds, bronchitis, diarrhea, arthritis, rheumatism, sore muscles, edema, intestinal conditions, headache

TRADITIONAL PREPARATION:

For diarrhea, bronchitis, intestinal conditions, and edema, make a decoction with a handful of chopped leaves and bark in 1-gallon water. Boil for 30 minutes. Strain, and sip throughout the day instead of water. **For arthritis, rheumatism, and sore muscles**, mash the leaves and apply directly to the affected area. The mashed leaves can also be used in a compress for wounds or headaches. **For bronchitis**, place 1 teaspoon dried leaves in 1/4 cup water and 1/2 teaspoon sugar. Bring to a boil and continue stirring until it reaches a syrup-like consistency. Drink by the spoonful.

Ixbut

With over 2,000 species of *Euphorbia*, ixbut stands out for its traditional medicinal use, particularly among the Maya. This plant is in the category of cactus and succulents, and it grows to

1 to 1.5 feet in height. The blooms are pale green in color, and the sap can be toxic. It is most commonly used in an infusion.

WHERE IT CAN BE FOUND:

Guatemala, Mexico, Honduras, Belize

PROPERTIES AND USE:

Antifungal, analgesic, antibacterial, antitumor, expectorant, antiparasitic, febrifuge, and used to treat poor lactation, stomach ailments, diarrhea, skin conditions, gonorrhea, constipation, warts, colic, sore muscles, rheumatism, bronchitis, oral infections, poor immune system function, respiratory conditions. In large doses, ixbut is emetic.

TRADITIONAL PREPARATION:

For all conditions, make an infusion of 3 dried leaves with stems in 1 cup boiling water. Make larger quantities and use as a rinse or bath **for skin conditions and for sore muscles. For warts**, apply the sap directly to the skin. **For oral infections**, dilute the sap with water, and use as a mouthwash.

DID YOU KNOW?

Many people have a hard time pronouncing ixbut, which is a Maya term. It is pronounced "ish-boot".

Jaboticaba

A small, plum-size fruit that is purple black in color, the jaboticaba fruit is both tasty and beneficial for medicinal use. This plant has been nicknamed the "anti-aging fruit" because it is high in antioxidants, which can help to slow down the signs of aging. The fruit is also good source of phenolic compounds, including anthocyanins. These might be helpful in the treatment of cancer.

This slow-growing tree produces salmon-colored leaves that turn green in maturity. When uncultivated, it produces fruit once or twice per year, but through proper cultivation, may produce fruit year-round. Other common names include *jabotica, jabuticaba,* Brazilian grape tree, *ybapuru, uva de árbol, guapuru, sabará,* and *hivapuru.* It is unusual in that its fruit grows directly on its trunk.

WHERE IT CAN BE FOUND:

Central America, Brazil, Paraguay, Bolivia, Argentina

PROPERTIES AND USE:

Astringent, anti-inflammatory, anti-aging, antitumor, detoxifier, and used to treat asthma, poor immune system function, ailments of the digestive tract, diarrhea, sore throat, low iron (especially in pregnant women)

TRADITIONAL PREPARATION:

For all conditions, eat 1/2 to 1 cup jaboticaba fruits per day. You may also use it as the basis for vinegars, liquor, juices, jelly, and jelly. **For diarrhea, low iron, asthma, and sore throat**, boil 2 teaspoons dried jaboticaba skins in 1 cup water for 5 minutes. Drink in one sitting. This decoction can also be gargled for sore throats.

DID YOU KNOW?

Because of its short shelf life, jaboticaba is mostly used domestically. Some predict that in its dried form, it will soon become widely available in Europe and North America as a follow up to popular açaí and guarana products.

Jackass Bitters

Growing from 3 to 14 feet, this herb has a few main stems with many branches. The leaves often have three distinct points, giving it its Spanish name, *tres puntas*. The leaves are bitter. Its flowers are yellow. Like all bitters, jackass bitters should not be consumed by pregnant women.

WHERE IT CAN BE FOUND:

Mexico, Caribbean, Central America, Northern South America to Brazil, Florida, Hawaii

Antifungal, antiparasitic, insecticidal, antimalarial, abortifacient, and used to treat head lice, sores, wounds, vaginal conditions, infections, skin conditions

TRADITIONAL PREPARATION:

For fungus, parasites, and infections, boil 1 fresh leaf per cup water for 10 minutes. Repeat up to three times per day. **For malaria**, drink 4 cups per day. **For external conditions**, boil 1 handful of jackass bitters leaves in 1-gallon water for 10 minutes. Allow to cool partially or completely, and then bathe the affected area. This liquid may be used on diseased houseplants or garden plants. It can also be used as a rinse for head lice, as a douche, or to bathe stubborn wounds or infections. Fresh, juiced leaves may also be used on **skin conditions and fungal infections**.

Jackfruit

A species of the mulberry family, this evergreen tree grows to 65 feet tall and produces the world's largest tree-borne fruit—up to 75 pounds each. The average fruits are 1 to 2 feet long, and up to 1 foot wide. The exterior is green yellow in color, with small, spiky knobs. The flesh is light yellow, with a banana-like flavor.

WHERE IT CAN BE FOUND:

Caribbean, Central America, India, Bangladesh, Nepal, Sri Lanka, Cambodia, Vietnam, Thailand, Philippines, Brazil, East Indies, Africa

PROPERTIES AND USE:

Anti-inflammatory, antibacterial, febrifuge, antivenomous, abortifacient (wood only), nervine, hypotensive, and used to treat constipation, diabetes, skin conditions, swollen glands, ulcers, poor immune system function, obesity, asthma, loss of memory, ADHD, wrinkles

TRADITIONAL PREPARATION:

For snakebites and skin conditions, chew the fruit, and pack into the wound. **For fevers, stress, hypertension, constipation, diabetes, swollen glands, ulcers, poor immune system function, obesity, loss of memory, and ADHD**, eat 1 cup of the fruit each day. **For asthma**, take 1 tablespoon jackfruit root extract twice per day. **To reduce fi ne lines and wrinkles**, spread the custard-like fruit's interior over the skin and leave on for 20 minutes. Repeat three times per week. This also works on other skin conditions.

DID YOU KNOW?

Rich in antioxidants and phytonutrients, jackfruit is being studied for its cancer-fighting properties.

Jícaro

This tree reaches up to 33 feet in height, and has twisted branches, and leathery, spatulate leaves. Its flowers are white or greenish, with dark purple stripes. The globose fruits, growing to a foot in diameter, have a smooth, fleshy green shell. In the Caribbean and Central America, where it is sometimes known as the calabash tree, it is used to ward off the evil eye.

WHERE IT CAN BE FOUND:

Caribbean, Central America, tropical South America, Florida

PROPERTIES AND USE:

Febrifuge, and used to treat whopping cough, tuberculosis, asthma, bronchitis, cough, flu, lung congestion, abscesses, mumps, earache, vomiting, slow labor, the removal of the placenta after childbirth

TRADITIONAL PREPARATION:

For all conditions, make an infusion by boiling a small handful of leaves in 1-gallon water. Strain, and allow to cool. Consume one to three cups per day. **For asthma, bronchitis, cough, flu, and lung congestion**, boil the inner pith of 1 mature fruit with 2 cups sugar and 2 quarts water for 30 minutes. Strain, and take by the spoonful six times per day.

DID YOU KNOW?

Jícaro gourds are used for containers, as well as in Maya rituals for good health and peaceful living. After removing the inner pith, the dried fruit is used as a vessel for many traditions, including the passing of atole—a popular hot corn beverage—at dinner parties. Drinking from the same gourd as your host generates good feelings and will ensure that you are invited and will gladly accept an invitation to return.

Lavender

The word lavender originates from the Latin root *lavare*, which means "to wash". This name is fitting because of the cleansing properties of lavender, which can be very beneficial for skin health. A beautifully fragrant shrub that grows to 6 feet in height, this purple flower has many other medicinal properties. It is one of the more common herbal remedies used today, and it can be purchased in many different forms.

WHERE IT CAN BE FOUND:

New York, Vermont, and cultivated worldwide

PROPERTIES AND USE:

Nervine, antidepressant, insecticidal, analgesic, decongestant, carminative, and used to treat morning sickness, motion sickness, skin conditions, wounds, diaper rash, bruises, insomnia, earache, headache

TRADITIONAL PREPARATION:

For all conditions, stir 1 teaspoon lavender buds in 1 cup boiling water. Strain, and drink in one sitting. Repeat up to twice per day to treat morning sickness and anxiety. Made in larger quantities, this infusion can be cooled and used as a rinse or bath. **For skin conditions, wounds, bruises, or headach**e, place a few drops highly concentrated essential oil in a carrier oil such as coconut or Macadamia nut oil and apply to the affected area. **For stress or insomnia**, place a drop of lavender essential oil in your palms, rub them together, and inhale deeply. Smooth your palms on your pillow to inhale the aromatic benefits as you sleep. Placing a few drops in a warm bath also melts away tension.

LAVENDER OIL
Makes 1 cup

This soothing oil can be rubbed on the chest to treat congestion. Applied to the temples, it treats headache. It's also great on diaper rash, bruises, and for massage. You will need an 8-ounce jar with lid and fi ne-mesh sieve or cheesecloth for this recipe. You also may want a large dropper bottle or assortment of smaller bottles for storage.

INGREDIENTS:

- 1/4 cup dried lavender buds

- 1 cup olive oil

INSTRUCTIONS:

- Place the buds in your jar with lid and pour in the oil to fill the jar.

- Tightly screw on the lid, and place on a windowsill too steep for six weeks. Shake the

- jar from time to time.

- After six weeks, store in a cool, dark area.

- To use, strain through cheesecloth or a fi ne-mesh sieve and pour into your dropper bottle(s).

USE:

This oil should keep for up to six months.

DID YOU KNOW?

There are actually 39 species of the lavender plant, and they offer similar medicinal benefits. *Lavandula angustifolia* is considered the official therapeutic grade species. It was first used by a French scientist René-Maurice Gattefossé in the early 1900's.

Lemongrass

This long, perennial grass grows in dense tufts of up to more than 6 feet tall. When growing in the wild, it may produce flowers, something it rarely does in cultivation. It is also known as fever grass. Due to its pleasant, lemony aroma, it is widely used in cooking.

WHERE IT CAN BE FOUND:

Caribbean, Southern India, Sri Lanka, Central America, tropical South America, Florida

PROPERTIES AND USE:

Antifungal, anti-inflammatory, antibacterial, febrifuge, expectorant, digestive, insecticidal, and is used to treat stomach cramps, backache, headache, sore throat, colitis, indigestion, gastrointestinal conditions, rheumatism, sore muscles, laryngitis, menstrual pain, nausea

TRADITIONAL PREPARATION:

For all conditions, cut off the root end of a lemongrass stalk, and remove any dry outer leaves. Gently bruise the root by lightly pounding it. Place in 1 cup boiling water, adding a cinnamon stick, a couple of cloves, and a squeeze of lime, if desired. **For ringworm**, mix 4 drops lemongrass essential oil with 10 drops jojoba oil. Apply directly to the affected area. **For**

sore throat or laryngitis, boil a few leaves in 1-gallon water. Remove from heat. Place a towel over the head, and inhale deeply. **For sore muscles**, apply the juice of the root and leaves directly to the affected area. You may also add a few drops lemon grass essential oil to lotion or massage oil. As an insecticide, place a few drops lemongrass essential oil in a spray bottle containing water. Spray throughout your house.

Licorice

Licorice is a perennial legume plant that can grow to 7 feet tall. It has pinnate leaves and pale blue to purple flowers up to 1/2 inch long. The fruit is an oblong pod containing several seeds. Fifty times sweeter than sugar, licorice root is used to treat a number of conditions. Though similar in flavor, it is not related to anise or fennel.

A relative, *Glycyrrhiza lepidota*, lives from Central Canada down through Texas and Virginia. It is used in the same manner.

WHERE IT CAN BE FOUND:

Asia, Northern Africa, Russia, Spain, Mexico, Central America, South America, Middle East, California, Nevada, Utah

PROPERTIES AND USE:

Antispasmodic, diuretic, anti-inflammatory, antibacterial, antiviral, hypertensive, emollient, expectorant, detoxifier, and treats prostate cancer, stomachache, sore throat, bronchitis, cough, respiratory infections, osteoarthritis, lupus, liver conditions, chronic fatigue syndrome, poor adrenal function, polycystic ovary syndrome, eczema, colic, heartburn, peptic ulcers, food poisoning, painful menstruation, mouth sores

TRADITIONAL PREPARATION:

For all conditions, boil 2 teaspoons dried licorice root in 1 cup water. Bring to a boil, and then remove from heat. Steep for 10 minutes. Strain before drinking. Except for those with high blood pressure, drink up to three cups per day. This decoction can be used as a mouthwash **to treat mouth sores**, and as a wash **for eczema or dry skin**.

DID YOU KNOW?

Most medicinal products and confections sold as licorice in the US contain no licorice.

Limon Indio

This shrubby, thorny tree up to 16 feet tall has a curved trunk and ovate leaves that resemble orange leaves. The flowers are yellowish-white, with a light purple margin. Flowers and fruit appear throughout the year. The green fruit is globose and 1 to 2 inches in diameter. It is seedier and more acidic than the limes sold in US grocery stories. In the US, it is known as Key lime.

WHERE IT CAN BE FOUND:

Mexico, Caribbean, Central America, tropical South America, India, Egypt, Texas, Florida, Georgia

PROPERTIES AND USE:

Febrifuge, vermifuge, antibacterial, diuretic, hepatoprotective, astringent, diuretic, antiseptic, tonic. Treats nausea, vomiting, cough, skin conditions, hemorrhoids, heart palpitations, body odor, rheumatism, arthritis, hair loss, halitosis, insomnia, insect bites, obesity, headache, stomach conditions, tired eyes.

TRADITIONAL PREPARATION:

To reduce fevers, place a 1-inch by 4-inch strip of bark in 1-quart water. Boil, covered, for 20 minutes. Remove from heat and allow too steep for 30 minutes. Drink instead of water until fever breaks. Drink 3 cups per day as a **diuretic, hepataprotective, tonic for nausea, vomiting, coughs, heart palpitations, body odor, rheumatism, arthritis, and for stomach conditions**. Drink 1 cup warm before bed for insomnia. Use cooled as a rinse for skin conditions, hair loss, and insect bites. Let sit for 15 minutes, and then rinse with cool water. **For nausea and vomiting**, combine 1 cup water, 10 drops lime juice, 1/2 teaspoon sugar, and 1/4 teaspoon baking soda. Drink in one serving. **As a vermifuge**, mix the juice of 1 lime with 1/4 cup extra-virgin olive oil. Drink in one sitting. **For coughs**, add 1/2 cup honey, the gel of 1 aloe Vera leaf, the juice of two limon indios, and 2 tablespoons chopped onions to a blender. Blend until smooth and administer 2 tablespoons per hour as needed. **For weight loss and to cleanse the system**, mix the juice of 1/2 lime and 1 teaspoon honey in 1 cup room temperature water. Drink first thing each morning. For halitosis, rinse with the juice of 1limon indio each morning and after each meal. **For headaches**, crush the leaves and apply directly to the forehead. **For tired eyes**, boil a handful of petals from a Rose of Castile in 1-liter water. Remove from heat and allow to cool. Add five drops limon indio juice and use as an eyewash.

DID YOU KNOW?

A quick fix x for insect bites is to rub the juice of a cut limon indio directly on the bite.

Linden Flower

Even though there are many superstitions and legends in Europe focused on linden flowers, they can be used for more than rituals, and are actually a great medicinal. This tree can grow as high as 120 feet tall, with fragrant, white-yellow flowers about 1/2 inch in width. The flowers grow in clusters, with each cluster on a long stalk. These flowers usually bloom between June and August, followed by small, round pea-sized seeds. Other names for the linden flower include bast tree, lime tree, and American basswood.

WHERE IT CAN BE FOUND:

Europe, Eastern US, Eastern Canada, Texas, South Carolina

PROPERTIES AND USE:

Hypotensive, decongestant, sedative, nervine, febrifuge, anti-inflammatory, diuretic, antispasmodic, and treats insomnia, diarrhea, sinus infections, headache, migraine, itchy skin, acne, sore throat

TRADITIONAL PREPARATION:

For all conditions, place 1 teaspoon dried linden flowers in 1 cup boiling water. You may repeat up to twice per day. Cooled, this infusion can be used as a rinse or bath **for itchy skin or acne**. Warm, it can be gargled **to treat sore throat**. The sapwood (inner bark of the tree) can also be used for medicine. Linden flower is available in a highly concentrated essential oil.

DID YOU KNOW?

In several European countries, linden was used to carve sacred works of art. People believed that the tree would bring prosperity and fertility, especially for people in love.

Liver Leaf

Liver leaf was a common plant in ancient times but fell into disuse in the late 1800s. Recently, its many health benefits and mild properties have been rediscovered. Liver leaf is sometimes called liverwort, though that name technically belongs to a different plant, *Marchantia polymorpha*. Liver leaf flowers early in the spring. It blooms among buds that are scaly in nature, the leftover growth from the previous year.

WHERE IT CAN BE FOUND:

Europe, Western Asia, Alabama, Arkansas, Connecticut, District of Columbia, Delaware, Florida, Georgia, Iowa, Illinois, Indiana, Kentucky, Massachusetts, Maryland, Maine, Michigan, Minnesota, Missouri, Mississippi, North Carolina, New Hampshire, New Jersey, New York, Ohio, Pennsylvania, Rhode Island, South Carolina, Tennessee, Virginia, Vermont, Wisconsin, West Virginia, Manitoba, New Brunswick, Nova Scotia, Ontario, Quebec

PROPERTIES AND USE:

Astringent, diuretic, detoxifier, hepatoprotective, and used to treat cough and other lung and respiratory problems including swollen mucous membranes

TRADITIONAL PREPARATION:

Liver leaf may be used as a tincture or tea, both of which can be beneficial **for liver cleansing**. The flowers and leaves can be used **for all respiratory ailments** and are especially good **for conditions that are slow healing**. When used in large doses, this remedy can be poisonous, so it is best used in small doses.

DID YOU KNOW?

Liver leaf gets its name from its dying leaves resembling the color and shape of a liver.

Loquat

This subtropical tree is part of the Rosaceae family, and it produces leaves, kernels, and fruit that can all be used for medicinal purposes. It is a rich source of a compound called amygdalin, which is thought to be beneficial for anti-cancer purposes.

Loquat is a shrub-like tree that has rich foliage and sweet, yellow fruit. The leaves have a serrated edge, and they are glossy and tough in nature. Other names include *nispero, pi pa ye, nespola giapponese*, Japanese medlar, Japanse plum tree, Chinese plum tree, *ameixa amarelle*, and *wollmispel*.

WHERE IT CAN BE FOUND:

Asia, South Africa, Australia, South America, India, Portugal, Spain, Germany, England, France, Italy, Central America, Caribbean, California, Florida, Georgia, Hawaii, Louisiana

PROPERTIES AND USE:

Expectorant, hypoglycemic, sedative, anti-inflammatory, antiviral, detoxifying, and treats respiratory ailments, coughs, obesity, vomiting, diarrhea, nausea, indigestion, poor immune system function, skin conditions

TRADITIONAL PREPARATION:

For all conditions, rub the fi ne hairs from the underside of the leaves. Wash the leaves and allow to dry completely. You may do this in an oven set to low, in the sun, or in a food dehydrator. Crush the dried leaves, and then make a decoction by boiling 1 tablespoon of the crushed leaf in 1-quart water for 15 to 20 minutes. Remove from heat, and steep for 30 minutes. Strain, and serve warm or cold, sweetened or unsweetened. Most conditions call for 1 glass per day. **For vomiting**, you may sip it until the symptoms subside. **For sore throats**, use the warm decoction as a gargle. As a rinse or bath for skin conditions, use it chilled. Topical creams or poultices are used

to treat rashes and other skin inflammation, as well as skin cancer.

DID YOU KNOW?

Loqat was discovered in 1690 by Engelbert Kaempfer, a medic and botanist in the Dutch East India Company. It was discovered in Japan in 1712, and then planted in England and Paris in the late 1700s. It has now spread all over the world.

Loroco

Loroco isn't widely known as a popular natural remedy outside of the Maya lands. The woody vine contains flower buds that bloom into beautiful white flowers. The flowers grow in clusters of about 25 flowers in each, and then will produce pods that change from a green to a dark brown color. Before the flowers bloom, the buds are often used in Central American cuisine.

In the US, it is available pickled in vinegar, brined, or frozen. It is not available fresh because the USDA found that the plant can sometimes carry *Diabrotica adelpha* beetles. Loroco used to be called Quilite, which means "edible herb".

WHERE IT CAN BE FOUND:

Central America

PROPERTIES AND USE:

Antispasmodic, nervine, stomachic, abortifacient, and treats poor immune system function

TRADITIONAL PREPARATION:

For all conditions, boil a small handful flowers in 1-gallon water. Strain, and drink 1 cup per day.

DID YOU KNOW?

The taste of loroco is somewhat mild, and can be compared to spinach, chard, or a mixture between squash and broccoli. Some people say that the taste has overtones of a nutty flavor. It is used in papusas, soups, salads, and sauces.

Macadamia

Leaves on the Macadamia tree are oblong and glossy, with wavy margins. The flowers are white in color, and often hidden among the leaves. The nuts are usually allowed to fall to the ground for harvesting, and then the hard, green outer layer and much harder inner layer are both removed. They are used medicinally, and for beauty treatments and in cooking. Macadamia nut oil has a good balance of both omega-3 and omega-6 essential fatty acids. Other names for Macadamia nuts include bush nut, bopple nut, and Australian nut.

WHERE IT CAN BE FOUND:

Caribbean, Australia, China, Indonesia, Thailand, Mexico, South Africa, Central America, Hawaii, Southern California, Florida

PROPERTIES AND USE:

Anti-aging, emollient, and used to treat high cholesterol, dandruff, dry skin

TRADITIONAL PREPARATION:

Often used as massage and beauty oil, Macadamia nut oil helps **to soften and soothe the skin and condition the hair**. In fact, it is frequently added to beauty products such as lip balm, lotion, body creams, scrubs, and hair care products. The oil can be used for cooking, as a substitute for any other type of cooking oil.

EMILIA'S MACADAMIA NUT OIL HAIR MASK

Despite the fact that she works outside in the sun and humidity of Guatemala, Emilia's silver hair is surprisingly healthy and shiny. This mask is why.

INGREDIENTS:

- 1 banana, mashed

- 1 tablespoon Macadamia nut oil

INSTRUCTIONS:

- Mix well to combine.

USE:

Apply directly to the hair. Allow to sit 1 hour, and then rinse.

EMILIA'S MACADAMIA NUT OIL FACIAL MASKS

Emilia Aguirre is a big fan of natural facial masks, and we asked her for her favorites for three different skin conditions.

FOR DRY SKIN

INGREDIENTS:

- 1 tablespoon banana

- 1 tablespoon honey

- 1 tablespoon ripe avocado

- 1 teaspoon Macadamia nut oil

INSTRUCTIONS:

- Combine the banana, honey, and avocado until smooth.

- Add the oil in a slow, steady stream to emulsify.

- Emilia wears this for 5 minutes. You can also use it in your hair.

FOR OILY SKIN

INGREDIENTS:

- 1 large strawberry, mashed

- 1 tablespoon banana

- 1 tablespoon honey

- 1 teaspoon Macadamia nut oil

INSTRUCTIONS:

- Combine the strawberry, banana, and honey until smooth.

- Add the oil in a slow, steady stream to emulsify.

- Wear for 5 minutes.

FOR INFLAMED OR IRRITATED SKIN

INGREDIENTS:

- 1 teaspoon turmeric

- 1 tablespoon Macadamia nut oil

INSTRUCTIONS:

- Mix well and apply to skin.

- Wear for 15 minutes.

DID YOU KNOW?

Even though Hawaii is often credited for the Macadamia nut industry, the cultivation of these nuts actually originated in Australia.

Madre De Cacao

We first encountered madre de cacao in Copán, where it was known as *mata ratón* or Gliricidia. This tree grows to just over 30 feet tall, and has a thin, dark brown trunk no more than a foot in diameter. The leaves are deciduous, divided into seven to 17 leaflets of 1 to 2.5 inches in length. The flowers range in color from white to bright pink. The pods are dark brown and grow up to 6 inches in length. We saw madre de cacao growing at ruin sites, in the forests and fields, and along the roadsides throughout our Central American trip.

WHERE IT CAN BE FOUND:

Mexico to Colombia, Venezuela to the Guianas, and tropical regions worldwide.

PROPERTIES AND USE:

Expectorant, insecticidal, vermicidal, sedative, and used to induce birth and for healing wounds, skin conditions, eye conditions, and diaper rash.

TRADITIONAL PREPARATION:

For all conditions, boil a 1-inch by 3-inch piece of bark in 1 cup water for 10 minutes. Drink in one sitting. This same decoction, when strained through cheesecloth until just liquid remains, is used to wash eyes. For wounds, skin conditions, and diaper rash, mash fresh leaves, and apply as a poultice.

Maitake

For many years, this fungus' health benefits were based on folklore. But modern researchers are finding that it does offer numerous health benefits. Maitake grows in clusters at the base of trees, with mushroom caps between 3/4 and 2 3/4 inches in width. The stalk becomes tougher in maturation. Other names include sheep's head, ram's head, and hen-of-the-woods.

WHERE IT CAN BE FOUND:

Temperate regions in Europe, Eastern Canada, the US (excluding the Pacific Northwest)

PROPERTIES AND USE:

Antitumor, hypoglycemic, antibacterial, hypotensive. Treats high cholesterol, diabetes, HIV, hepatitis, poor immune system function, hay fever, obesity, chronic fatigue syndrome, infertility caused by polycystic ovary syndrome, and the negative side effects of chemotherapy and other drugs from the treatment of cancer.

TRADITIONAL PREPARATION:

For all conditions, eat maitake mushrooms raw, sautéed, or in soups. You may also prepare an infusion by using 1 teaspoon maitake powder per cup boiling water. Maitake is widely available in capsule and liquid form. Administer 3 to 7 grams per day.

DID YOU KNOW?

The word maitake is Japanese and means "dancing mushroom". Ancient Japanese people were said to dance when these mushrooms were discovered, because they were very valuable and rare. At the time, the mushrooms were worth their weight in silver.

Mamey Sapote

As an ancient Aztec remedy, mamey sapote has also gained popularity throughout North and South America. It is an ornamental evergreen tree that grows to 140 feet high. The fruit is meaty with orange flesh, brown skin, and a black pit in its center. The taste of the fruit is earthy and sweet, with fragrant flavors. The flesh is non-fibrous, which has earned it the nickname "orange avocado". Other common names include mamey Colorado and *sapote*.

WHERE IT CAN BE FOUND:

Central America, South America, Caribbean, Australia, Florida, and tropical countries worldwide

PROPERTIES AND USE:

Antitumor, antiseptic, aphrodisiac, antifungal, hypotensive, antispasmodic, anti-inflammatory, and used to treat rheumatism, arthritis, sore muscles, high cholesterol, indigestion, toothache, eye and ear conditions, skin conditions, epilepsy, diarrhea, hair loss, poor immune system function, venereal disease, headache

TRADITIONAL PREPARATION:

The Aztecs roasted the seeds, and then crushed them into powder for use in a poultice. They also extracted the oil from the seeds and used it **as a hair treatment and to treat skin conditions, earache, and eye infection. For all conditions**, eat the fruit raw. You may also create a decoction by placing 3 tablespoons of the dried herb in 1-quart cold water. Cover, and cook over low heat. Simmer for 45 minutes. Strain, and drink 2 cups per day. **For inflammation, rheumatism, arthritis, and sore muscles**, crush the leaves and apply directly to the affected area. Repeat for three days, or until the symptoms subside.

DID YOU KNOW?

The flesh of the mamey sapote fruit is salmon in color. It tastes similar to a pumpkin or sweet potato, with hints of honey or cherry.

Man Strength

Man, strength is revered throughout the Caribbean, where it is also known as fourman strength. Popular in the root tonics served throughout the islands, it is said to make a man feel invincible. It also helps with male impotence. Its medicinal properties are not limited to men, however, as it is also prescribed for removing clots and discharge after childbirth, for postpartum depression, and as a uterine tonic. It is a small, woody herb that grows in wet areas and stands erectly. It has very small evergreen leaves, and round, thin stems. It is a bitter and should therefore not be consumed by pregnant women.

WHERE IT CAN BE FOUND:

Caribbean, Central America, tropical South America, Miami-Dade County Florida

PROPERTIES AND USE:

Stomachic, tonic, aphrodisiac, analgesic, and is used to treat diabetes, postpartum depression, blood clots after childbirth, edema, skin conditions, male impotence, urinary tract infections

TRADITIONAL PREPARATION:

As a stomachic, tonic, aphrodisiac, and to treat diabetes, urinary tract infections, and post-childbirth symptoms, a handful of roots is soaked in 1-liter rum and taken as a shot twice per day. **For skin conditions**, boil a small handful of roots in 1-gallon water for 30 minutes. Remove from heat and allow to soak overnight. Strain, and use as a wash.

Mango Bark

Mango indica Linn. is the world's largest fruit tree, growing to 100 feet high, with a trunk up to 20 feet in circumference. The bark, roots, flowers, leaves, and fruit all possess different and myriad health benefits. Don Alejandro León Recino, a Maya healer we met in Nuevo Esperanza, Honduras, spoke to us at length about the health benefits of the bark. It's one of his go-to treatments.

WHERE IT CAN BE FOUND:

India, Caribbean, Central America, South America, Southeast Asia, Australia, West Africa, Florida, Hawaii

PROPERTIES AND USE:

Astringent, anti-inflammatory, stomachic, antiparasitic, antibiotic, febrifuge, hypotensive, and used to treat indigestion, diarrhea, parasitic skin conditions, vomiting, nausea, syphilis, bleeding wounds, ulcers, heavy menstruation, diabetes. It also treats a condition known as having too much "heat" in the system.

TRADITIONAL PREPARATION:

For all conditions, boil three 4-inch by 6-inch pieces of mango bark in 1-gallon water for 30 minutes. Strain, and drink in place of water until symptoms subside. **For heavy menstruation or too much "heat" in the system**, juice a 4-inch by 6-inch piece of mango bark. Add to 1-liter water. Administer by the teaspoonful until symptoms subside.

Mangosteen

The Mangosteen is a slow-growing tree with dark brown, flaking skin and fruit that is about the size of an apple or a peach. It has a hard rind, with soft fruit inside. To eat the fruit, it is necessary to open it up by twisting the outside or pressing firmly until it breaks. The rind contains tannins, which have been associated with anti-inflammatory benefits. Another common name for mangosteen juice is *xango* and queen of fruits.

WHERE IT CAN BE FOUND:

Indonesia, Malaysia, Southeast and South Asia

PROPERTIES AND USE:

Anti-inflammatory, anti-allergen, antibacterial, antiseptic, antitumor, antifungal, antiviral, hypotensive, tonic, and used to treat urinary tract infections, thrush, gonorrhea, diarrhea, dysentery, difficult menstruation, rheumatism, arthritis, sore muscles, high cholesterol, anemia

TRADITIONAL PREPARATION:

For all conditions, eat raw, juiced, or make into a jam. The rind can be made into an infusion **to treat gonorrhea, bladder infections, and diarrhea**. And ointment **for rashes** can be made by grinding the rind.

MANGOSTEEN JELLY

This sweet treat contains medicinal mangosteen, as well as lime, which aids in the healing of wounds, prevents damage to the eyes, maintains dental health, and helps with digestion and peptic ulcers. A natural antibiotic, it is also used for weight reduction and the treatment of cysts.

INGREDIENTS:

- 1/3 cup sugar

- 1/3 cup water

- 1 cup mangosteen pulp or puree

- 2 tablespoons lime juice

- 1 tablespoon pectin

INSTRUCTIONS:

- Make a simple syrup by cooking the sugar and water over medium heat until syrupy.

- Stir in the mangosteen, lime juice, and pectin.

- When the mixture reaches your desired consistency, cool and then store in a jar with lid.

USE:

This jelly is wonderful when added to your favorite smoothie

Maracujá

Maracujá, known in the US as passionflower, is a hardy, woody vine that grows to more than 30 feet tall and has tendrils. It has large, white flowers with pink or purple centers. It produces the passion fruit, which is a delicious form of nutrition in tropical regions.

WHERE IT CAN BE FOUND:

Eastern and Southern Australia, Southern Africa, New Zealand, Caribbean, Florida, Georgia, Hawaii

PROPERTIES AND USE:

Analgesic, nervine, anti-inflammatory, antispasmodic, sedative, antibacterial, diuretic, aphrodisiac, hypotensive, vermifuge, and is used to treat depression, epilepsy, Parkinson's disease, headache, bruises, cough, heart disease, alcoholism, insomnia, nicotine addiction

TRADITIONAL PREPARATION:

For all conditions, eating the fruit is advised. **As a nervine, sedative, and to treat water retention, epilepsy, Parkinson's disease, heart disease, alcoholism, and nicotine addiction**, boil 3 leaves in 1 cup water. Drink while warm and repeat three times per day. **For headaches**, apply the leaves or fruit pulp as a poultice. **For coughs**, boil 1 fruit in 1/2 cup water and 2 teaspoons sugar until syrupy. Administer 1 teaspoon every hour until symptoms subside.

Marañon

Marañon, or cashew, in English, is widely known as a nut. It is, however, a seed—that of the *Anacardium occidentale* L. tree, an evergreen that grows to more than 40 feet tall. The fruit, a pseudocarp or false fruit, is oval or pear shaped and often called a cashew apple. It ripens into a yellow and/or red color and smells and tastes sweet. The true fruit is a drupe growing at the end of the cashew apple. It resembles a boxing glove. Within this is one seed, or the so-called cashew nut.

WHERE IT CAN BE FOUND:

Caribbean, Central America, South America, India, China, East Africa

PROPERTIES AND USE:

Decongestant, digestive, stimulant, diuretic, febrifuge, hypotensive, purgative, tonic, antibacterial, aphrodisiac, hypoglycemic, antimalarial, and used to treat wounds, "heat" in the system, cough, diarrhea, dysentery, colic

TRADITIONAL PREPARATION:

For all conditions, boil a large handful of leaves and branches in 1-gallon water. Strain, and drink 1/2 cup per day as necessary. You may also juice 2 fruits and drink throughout the day. **For too much "heat" in the system, fever, hypertension, and high blood sugar**, boil a 1-inch by 1-inch piece of bark and a leaf for 20 minutes. Remove from heat and steep for 20 minutes. Strain, and drink 1 cup two times per day. **For colic**, administer 2 teaspoons per day.

Marigold

Though you might admire marigold in a flowerbed or decorative pot, you might not realize its great healing potential. Other plants that are referred to as marigold have some of the same medicinal benefits. An example is *Calendula offiinalis*, found in the Mediterranean, Western Europe, Southwestern Asia, India, Central America, and parts of the US and Canada. This marigold is an erect annual herb up to 3 feet tall, with pinnate leaves and aromatic flowers that grow in solitary, gold-colored heads. *Tagetes erecta* L. is also known as Aztec marigold, and despite its being native to the Americas, African marigold.

WHERE IT CAN BE FOUND:

Mexico, Central America, Caribbean, Peru, Ecuador, Argentina, Venezuela, India, South Africa, Arkansas, California, Connecticut, Florida, Kentucky, Louisiana, Massachusetts, Maryland, Missouri, North Carolina, New Jersey, New York, Ohio, Oklahoma, Pennsylvania, South Carolina, Utah, Virginia, Quebec

PROPERTIES AND USE:

Carminative, digestive, diuretic, stimulant, emmenagogue, sedative, stomachic, febrifuge, and treats indigestion, colic, constipation, cough, dysentery, insect bites or stings, sores and ulcers of the skin, burns, wounds, headache, sore eyes, malaise, flu

TRADITIONAL PREPARATION:

To treat fever, colic, stomach cramps, and gas, steep 3 flower heads in 1 cup hot water for 10 minutes. **For colic and children suffering from malaise, diarrhea, fever, colds, and flu**, boil an entire plant in 2 gallons water for 10 minutes. Use as a bath. This is also used as a rinse or bath **for skin conditions, burns, and wounds**. **For insect bites or stings**, rub the head of a marigold on the affected area. **For sore eyes**, place 3 marigold heads in 1-gallon distilled water for at least 1 hour. Use as an eyewash.

DID YOU KNOW?

Marigold is being studied for its potential cholesterol lowering properties

Milk Thistle

Milk thistles can grow to 12 to 79 inches tall, and have an overall conical shape. They are hairless, shiny green, with milk-white veins. The flower heads are 4 to 12 cm long and wide, of red-purple colour. They flower from June to August in the North or December to February in the Southern Hemisphere (summer through autumn).

WHERE IT CAN BE FOUND:

Originally a native of Southern Europe through to Asia, it is now found throughout the world.

PROPERTIES AND USE:

Liver cleanse, aids digestion, lowers cholesterol and helpful for hepatitis and diabetes. It boosts the immune system.

TRADITIONAL PREPARATION:

Can be used in pill form, as a tea and oral tinctures.

Mint

Mint isn't just pleasant in a cup of tea. It's highly medicinal, too. Even just the aroma rising from your mug can soothe an upset stomach and open sinuses before the cup even touches your lips. This variety of mint grows to 2 feet tall, with short-stalked, lance-shaped leaves that are bright green and serrated. *Mentha spicata* is also called *hierbabuena* or spearmint.

WHERE IT CAN BE FOUND:

Native to Europe, it now also grows in Southwest Asia, Mexico, Central America, and every US state except North Dakota

PROPERTIES AND USE:

Analgesic, antitumor, antifungal, antibacterial, antispasmodic, stimulant, insecticide, diuretic, decongestant, hepatoprotective, carminative, antiseptic, stomachic, febrifuge, tonic. Treats colds, bronchitis, sore throat, headache, sinusitis, nausea, morning sickness, motion sickness, sore muscles, sciatica, backache, irritable bowel syndrome, indigestion, cramps, halitosis, painful menstruation, bronchitis, rheumatism.

TRADITIONAL PREPARATION:

For all conditions, you may eat the leaves raw. You can also make an infusion by pouring 1 cup boiling water over 1 small sprig of spearmint. **For sinus congestion**, place a towel over the head, and inhale the steam from the infusion. **For headaches and sore muscles**, apply spearmint oil directly on the affected area. **For halitosis**, chew raw leaves, or use the infusion as a mouthwash.

Moho

Moho is a shrubby, tropical evergreen tree that reaches more than 20 feet and is often grown as an ornamental plant. But it possesses many medicinal properties, as well.

Moho produces pale yellow or white spikes that are cord-like and flower. It is in the pepper family, and all its plant parts smell and taste spicy. For this reason, it's often used as a substitute for pepper and other condiments. It is also known as *matico*.

WHERE IT CAN BE FOUND:

Southern Mexico, Caribbean, tropical South America, Asia, Polynesia, Florida, Hawaii

PROPERTIES AND USE:

Antibacterial, antifungal, antiviral, carminative, antihemorrhagic, antiseptic, antitumor. Treats digestive conditions, wounds, skin conditions, uterine conditions, colds, cough, flu, throat cancer, uterine cancer, yeast infection, vomiting.

TRADITIONAL PREPARATION:

Moho can be purchased in capsule or extract form. The capsules are good as a supplement, and the extract can be used externally on **skin conditions. For wounds**, crush or powder the leaves, and apply directly to the affected area. **For all conditions**, make an infusion by boiling 3 leaves in 1-liter of water for 20 minutes. Remove from heat, and steep for 20 minutes. Drink 3 cups per day.

UTERINE CANCER VAGINAL STEAM BATH
Makes 1 treatment

Vaginal steam baths, called bajos, are used to treat a variety of conditions, from fi broids to cancer. For this treatment, you will need a chair with a slatted seat, a heavy blanket, and a large pot, bowl, or tub.

You will also need to remove your clothes from the waist down. If you are prone to cold feet, leave your socks on.

INGREDIENTS:

- 1 tablespoon moho powder

- 1 tablespoon dried fenugreek

- 1 tablespoon dried calendula

- 1/2 tablespoon sulfur

INSTRUCTIONS:

- Add all ingredients to 1-gallon boiling water.

- Allow to cool slightly, and then place the mixture under your chair. Making sure the steam is hot but not too hot, sit on the chair and use the blanket to cover the upper body and to tent the steam.

- Sit for 20 minutes, and then lie down and rest under dry, heavy bedding for 1 hour.

USE:

It is recommended to do this vaginal steam bath two times per week.

DID YOU KNOW?

Some countries view moho as a noxious weed, because the seeds can be scattered easily and spread quickly. When this happens, it can begin to choke out the vegetation native to the area.

Moringa

Moringa is a drought-resistant, fast-growing tree with many uses. In fact, practitioners of Ayurvedic medicine have said that this tree can be used to prevent and treat over 300 diseases.

All parts of the plant can be used for medicinal purposes, including the root, seeds, flowers, bark, and leaves. It has been nicknamed "the miracle plant" because of all of the medical and nutritional benefits that can be gained from its use. Other names include *kelor* tree, *malunggay*, drumstick tree, horseradish tree, Ben nut tree, and Indian horseradish.

WHERE IT CAN BE FOUND:

India, Africa, East Indies, Central America, tropical South America, Sri Lanka, India, Mexico, Malabar, Malaysia, Philippines

PROPERTIES AND USE:

Febrifuge, anti-inflammatory, hypotensive, hypoglycemic, hepatoprotective, antiparasitic, antibacterial, antifungal. Treats gout, insect bites, wounds, poor circulation, high cholesterol, diarrhea, gastric ulcers, colds, ear infection, bronchitis, spleen conditions, poor lactation.

TRADITIONAL PREPARATION:

To improve the flow and quality of breast milk, juice the moringa flower. Consume 1/2 to 1 cup per day. **For all other conditions**, make an infusion with 3 tablespoons dried moringa flower added to 1-liter boiling water. Strain, and drink in place of water. You may also make an infusion by grinding the dried leaves of 3 stalks and adding it to 1-liter boiling water. Cooled, this can be used as a **wash for fungal or bacterial infections**. You may wish to add lemon and sweetener. **For spleen and liver conditions**, eat the raw pods. This is also great for treating parasites. **For insect bites, fungal, or bacterial infections**, apply the extract directly to the skin. **For bleeding wounds**, apply a fresh leaf poultice.

DID YOU KNOW?

The leaves of the moringa tree are highly nutritious, with more vitamin C than oranges, more calcium than milk, more protein than yogurt, more potassium than bananas, and more vitamin A than carrots.

Mugwort

Even though it is sometimes overlooked for other more common herbal remedies, traditional Eastern and Western herbalists still use mugwort because of the many health benefits that it can offer. Mugwort is a tall plant, which can grow as high as 3 feet or more. The leaves have a purplish hue with a tint of dark green on the surface and are smooth and covered with a cottony texture underneath. The flowers grow in clusters, and they are yellowish or whitish-green in color. Other common names include St. John's plant or wormwood. Sometimes it is burned during ceremonies.

WHERE IT CAN BE FOUND:

North Africa; Europe; Turkey; Northern Iraq; Iran; Siberia; all of Canada except Yukon Territory, Northwest Territories, and Nunavut Territory; and US states except California, Nevada, Utah, Arizona, New Mexico, Colorado, Texas, Oklahoma, Nebraska, South Dakota, North Dakota, Wyoming

PROPERTIES AND USE:

Nervine, carminative, stimulant, tonic, diuretic, diaphoretic, emmenagogue, antispasmodic, antibacterial, antifungal, antidepressant, and treats addiction, insomnia, irritability, fertility issues, diarrhea, vomiting, constipation, fibromyalgia, irritable bowel syndrome, indigestion, irregular menstruation, stiff muscles, sciatica, epilepsy, rashes from plants or insects

TRADITIONAL PREPARATION:

For stress, insomnia, irritability, and epilepsy, pour 1 cup boiling water over 1 teaspoon dried mugwort leaves, 1 teaspoon dried chamomile flowers, and 1 teaspoon dried woodruff leaves. Steep for 10 to 15 minutes, and then strain. You may use passionflower and lobelia instead of chamomile and woodruff. **For rashes from plants or insects**, macerate the leaves in a small bowl with a tiny bit of water. Once the leaves are mushy, apply them directly to the affected area. You may also crush them with a mortar and pestle, or with the edge of a knife. **For muscle stiffness or sciatica pain**, combine mugwort with vinegar and agrimony, and apply topically.

DID YOU KNOW?

Mugwort is one of the most common ingredients in sleep pillows, and it has been said that it can help the person to experience lucid dreams.

Myrrh

Popular ancient texts refer to the use of myrrh, and given its medicinal properties, it's easy to see why. Myrrh is a shrub or small tree with thorny branches. The prized resin seeps from fissures in the bark. As it begins to harden, it is harvested for use in natural remedies. The aroma of myrrh is warm, spicy, and balsamic.

WHERE IT CAN BE FOUND:

Middle East, Africa, cultivated in parts of Central America and India

PROPERTIES AND USE:

Antifungal, astringent, antiseptic, expectorant, sedative, decongestant, anti-inflammatory, stomachic, emmenagogue. Treats cancer, skin conditions, oral health conditions, high cholesterol, wounds, laryngitis, sore throat.

TRADITIONAL PREPARATION:

The resin is used **for most remedies**. It can be gargled with water **to clear up laryngitis or to soothe a sore throat. For topical application**, dilute with a carrier oil before applying directly to a wound or skin irritation. Myrrh is most often sold as a tincture, but it can also be purchased as an essential oil. Sometimes it is available in a capsule or tea.

DID YOU KNOW?

Myrrh is traditionally known as one of the three gifts from the Three Magi in the Bible story, and it was given as an anesthetic to Jesus during his crucifixion. It was also used in ancient Egypt for embalming and for religious rituals.

Nettle

It might seem counter-intuitive to reach for a natural remedy from a plant that might hurt you, but don't be nervous about the nettle's "sting". You can find it in a usable form, so that you can enjoy the natural benefits without the skin irritation that can come from touching the plant. Nettle usually grows to about 3 feet tall and has soft green leaves that grow on a wiry stem. The flowers are dense and numerous, and they are usually brownish or greenish in color. Other names include stinging nettle, burn hazel, burn week, burn nettle, and common nettle.

WHERE IT CAN BE FOUND:

Northern Africa, Asia, Europe, every US state except Arkansas, every Canadian province except Nunavut

PROPERTIES AND USE:

Anti-allergen, diuretic, anti-inflammatory, aphrodisiac, antihemorrhagic, and treats hair loss, female hormonal imbalance, PMS, adrenal fatigue, kidney conditions, benign prostatic hyperplasia, urinary tract infections, osteoarthritis, diabetes, diarrhea, skin conditions, anemia, gout

TRADITIONAL PREPARATION:

For gout, juice the leaves and stems. Administer several teaspoons per day. **For all other conditions**, place 1 tablespoon chopped fresh nettle in 3 cups boiling water. Steep for 20 minutes. Strain, and drink hot or cold. Use as a rinse for hair loss.

DID YOU KNOW?

When your skin touches stinging nettle, there are bristles of histamine that cause a stinging burn to irritate your skin. Only certain types of nettle sting, so there are some plants that can be touched without risk of skin irritation.

Noni

Noni is an evergreen tree that can grow in a variety of environments, including sandy or rocky shores and shady forests. It takes about a year and a half before the plant reaches maturity, and then it produces between eight and 17 pounds of fruit per month. The leaves are large and dark green in color, with deep veins. Flowers bloom throughout the year and are small and clustered. The fruit is a yellow-white color as it ripens, with a lot of seeds, bitter taste, and pungent odor. Other common names for noni include beach mulberry, cheese fruit, Indian mulberry, and great morinda.

WHERE IT CAN BE FOUND:

Native to Australia and Southeast Asia, and grown in tropical areas worldwide

PROPERTIES AND USE:

Hypotensive, emmenagogue, anti-inflammatory, analgesic, hypotensive, febrifuge, antispasmodic, antidepressant, sedative. Treats PMS, vaginal discharge after childbirth, sore muscles, arthritis, infection, sores, burns, wounds, migraine, constipation, cancer, cataracts, smallpox, spleen conditions, colic, asthma, gastric ulcers, cough, liver disease, cataracts, AIDS, sprains, poor digestion, circulation problems, atherosclerosis, nausea, difficult childbirth, memory loss, drug addiction.

TRADITIONAL PREPARATION:

The fruit can be eaten, or it can be turned into a powder or juice. Medicinal remedies can be created from most parts of the plant, including the roots, bark, stems, flowers, leaves, and fruit. Most often, people use Noni extract that is taken orally. The bark has historically been used **to aid childbirth**. The leaves are often used as a poultice **to relieve arthritic pain and swelling**. When used as a juice or tea, it is usually combined with other ingredients to improve the taste. Two ounces of juice is recommended per day. **For all conditions**, pour 1 cup boiling water over 1 teaspoon dried noni leaf. Strain before drinking. Consume up to four cups per day.

DID YOU KNOW?

The smell of noni plants attracts fruit bats, who disperse the seeds as they fly.

Nopal

This prickly powerhouse is known by many names to many people: tuna, *scoggineal, opuntia, cochineal* cactus, prickly pear, white *tungi*, and many others. Growing to 10 feet and having large, thorny pads, this cactus has red flowers and ellipsoid, red-pink fruits.

WHERE IT CAN BE FOUND:

Pacific Islands, China, Mexico, Caribbean, Florida, Hawaii

PROPERTIES AND USE:

Anti-inflammatory, hypotensive, febrifuge, tonic, digestive, and used to treat skin ulcers, hair loss, difficult childbirth, obesity, high cholesterol, headache, diabetes, urinary tract infections, arthritis

TRADITIONAL PREPARATION:

For headaches and fevers, carefully peel a pad. Slice it in half lengthwise and tie it around the head. **For hypertension and fever**, boil 1 pad in 3 cups water for 5 minutes. Drink 1 cup before each meal. **For urinary tract infections**, crush and soak 5 pads in 1-gallon water overnight. Drink 1 to 2 cups per day until symptoms subside. **For difficult childbirth**, drink 1 cup juice. **For arthritis**, peel, steam, and chill pads, eat a pad per day. For skin ulcers, slice a pad in half lengthwise and apply to the affected area.

NOPAL HAIR MASK
Makes 1 treatment

The same qualities that allow the nopal to survive the scorching sun can rejuvenate and hydrate your hair. This mask is used for conditioning, as well as for hair loss and as a relaxer.

INSTRUCTIONS:

- Peel and mash the fruit.

- Spread it on clean hair.

- Cover with a shower cap or plastic wrap for 1 hour, and then rinse.

USE:

Repeat each week as necessary.

Nutmeg

The nutmeg tree produces egg-shaped seeds that are about an inch long and are dried before being ground into the common cooking spice. The trees don't start producing until seven to nine years after planting. Full production isn't achieved until the tree is 20 years old. Other common names include *pipo*, *mace*, *musketbaum*, and *myristica*.

WHERE IT CAN BE FOUND:

South Pacific Islands, Caribbean, Sri Lanka, Indonesia

PROPERTIES AND USE:

Carminative, sedative, antidepressant, hypotensive, hepatoprotective, aphrodisiac, analgesic, antibacterial, nervine. Treats diarrhea, stomach conditions, insomnia, memory loss, arthritis, rheumatism, poor circulation, hormone imbalance, toothache, Alzheimer's disease, skin conditions, wounds

TRADITIONAL PREPARATION:

For insomnia, add a pinch of nutmeg to a warm glass of milk. **For skin conditions and wounds**, make a rub with raw honey and nutmeg. **For toothache**, add a pinch of nutmeg to 1 cup hot water. Use as a gargle. **For all conditions**, add nutmeg to your diet. In the Caribbean, equal parts nutmeg and egg yolk are combined and applied to **infected umbilical cords**.

DID YOU KNOW?

In ancient times, Greek and Roman civilizations made a brain tonic out of nutmeg.

Oak

Perhaps no tree is as steeped in myth as the mighty oak. Known as the "tree of life" to the tribes inhabiting Oregon and Northern California, *Quercus kelloggii* Newberry was used as food, medicine, dye, and for construction. Its acorns were a staple, and are still used today in soups, breads, patties, and herbal cures. This species of oak goes by the common name California black oak or Kellogg oak. A close relative of *Quercus velutina*, the black oak found in the Eastern and Central United States, *Quercus kelloggii* Newberry grows to 80 feet in height and has a trunk that grows to 4.5 feet in diameter.

WHERE IT CAN BE FOUND:

Oregon, California

PROPERTIES AND USE:

Digestive, febrifuge, anti-inflammatory, and treats diarrhea, colds, cough, bronchitis, itchy skin, indigestion, bowel conditions

TRADITIONAL PREPARATION:

For indigestion and bowel conditions, make "charcoal soup" by charring the bark over an open flame. Boil in water, and strain before drinking. **For all other conditions**, place a large handful of green bark in 1-gallon water. Boil for 30 minutes, and then remove from heat and steep for 30 minutes. Strain, and sip a cup or two throughout the day. Cooled, this can be used as a rinse or bath **to treat itchy skin or inflammation**.

Ojushte

Also known as *masica, mojote, capomo,* breadnut, *ramón,* and Maya nut, *Brosimum alicastrum* is a very large evergreen tree that grows to 130 feet tall. It has a large seed, often mistakenly called a nut, that is covered by a thin, orange, citrus-flavored skin. It was significant to the ancient Maya both for nutrition and for spiritual use. Today, it is milled into flour and used as a coffee substitute.

WHERE IT CAN BE FOUND:

Mexico, Caribbean, Central America, Amazon

PROPERTIES AND USE:

Stimulant, anti-inflammatory, anti-aging, tonic, laxative, and is used for asthma, anemia, rheumatism, cough, colds, poor milk production, diabetes, tuberculosis, bronchitis, poor kidney function, lung infections

TRADITIONAL PREPARATION:

For all conditions, administer by the teaspoonful the latex from the leaves. One to 2 teaspoons per day is typical. **For diabetes, cough, tuberculosis, and bronchitis**, boil 1 small handful of the leaves and bark in 1-gallon water for 1 hour. Strain, and consume 1 cup per day. **For asthma and anemia**, take 1 teaspoon of ojushte tincture per day. **For coughs and**

colds, boil 1 leaf, 1/2 cup water, and 1 teaspoon sugar until syrupy. Drink 1 teaspoon per day.

OJUSHTE TINCTURE
Makes 2 cups

If you cannot find fresh ojushte root and bark, substitute 1 teaspoon dried. You will need a 16-ounce canning jar with lid for this recipe.

INGREDIENTS:

- 1 1/4 cups chopped ojushte root and bark

- 2 cups 100-proof vodka

INSTRUCTIONS:

- Pack a jar three-quarters full of ojushte root and bark.

- Pour in 100-proof vodka to fill the jar. Tightly screw on the lid, and place on a windowsill too steep for six weeks.

- After six weeks, store in a cool, dark area. The tincture should keep for up to three years.

USE:

For a pick-me-up, asthma, and anemia, take 1 teaspoon per day.

DID YOU KNOW?

One mature ojushte tree can produce up to 800 pounds of food per year. It can live for more than 100 years.

Orange Jessamine

Also known as orange jasmine or mock orange, orange jessamine is used in aromatherapy and in the creation of cosmetics and perfumes. It is a tropical evergreen shrub that grows to more than 20 feet tall and produces clusters of white, jasmine-scented flowers. Its fruits are small ovals orange to red in color.

WHERE IT CAN BE FOUND:

Australia, Asia, Mexico, Central America, Caribbean, Florida, Hawaii

PROPERTIES AND USE:

Stimulant, decongestant, astringent, and used to treat diarrhea, dysentery, wounds, rheumatism, sore muscles, venereal disease

TRADITIONAL PREPARATION:

For all conditions, pour 1 cup boiling water over 2 teaspoons dried flowers. Steep for 5 to 8 minutes. Strain, and serve warm. Drink up to 3 cups per day. Cooled, the infusion is used as a wash **for wounds**. **For rheumatism and sore muscles**, dry the flowers, and then crush into a powder. Apply as a poultice.

Oregano

The smell of oregano is often associated with pizza and pasta dishes and adding this herb to popular foods is a great way to boost your health. Oil of oregano is a powerful extract to boost immune system function and treats a variety of health issues. It is a perennial herb that grows to 2.5 feet tall. Its leaves and purple flowers are used for medicinal purposes. It is sometimes called wild marjoram.

WHERE IT CAN BE FOUND:

Mediterranean, India, Baltic states, Central Asia, Mexico, Central America, Arkansas, California, Delaware, Illinois, Massachusetts, Maryland, Michigan, North Carolina, New Jersey, New York, Ohio, Oregon, Pennsylvania, Virginia, Vermont, Washington, British Columbia, Nova Scotia, Ontario, Prince Edward Island, Quebec

PROPERTIES AND USE:

Antiparasitic, antiviral, antibacterial, antifungal, anti-inflammatory, analgesic, expectorant, tonic, anti-allergen, insecticide. Strengthens the immune system and can be an effective defense treatment if a virus is in the early stages. Strong antibacterial properties can knock out infections anywhere in the body. Treats respiratory conditions, bronchitis, sinus infections, urinary tract infections, skin conditions, burns, headache, dandruff, gum disease, sore muscles, varicose veins, asthma, croup, heartburn, halitosis

TRADITIONAL PREPARATION:

For all conditions, pour 1 cup boiling water over 1 teaspoon dried oregano. Strain before drinking. Use as a mouthwash **for gum disease and halitosis**. When oil of oregano is applied on the skin, it must be heavily diluted with a carrier oil **to avoid skin irritation**. The oil also helps with acne, and you can add a drop or two to facial cleanser **to avoid breakouts**.

DID YOU KNOW?

Oil of oregano is so concentrated that it takes about 100 pounds of fresh oregano leaves to make one pound of oil.

OREGANO OIL
Makes 1 cup

Oil of oregano is the oil extracted from the oregano leaves. This is an infused oil, great for cooking or topical application. You will need an 8-ounce container with lid for this recipe. An empty oil bottle works well for storage.

INGREDIENTS:

- 1 cup dried oregano

- 1 cup extra virgin olive of grape seed oil

INSTRUCTIONS:

- Heat the oil over low heat for about 2 minutes. Add the oregano and stir.

- Pour into a jar and tightly screw on the lid. Store in a cool, dark, place for 2 weeks.

- After 2 weeks, strain the oil through cheesecloth or a fine-mesh sieve. Pour into an empty oil bottle, from which you can easily fill dropper bottles as needed.

USE:

Take 1 teaspoon per day as a tonic, and to treat parasites and allergies. Apply topically to treat skin conditions, burns, headache, dandruff, sore muscles, and varicose veins.

Osha Root

A member of the apiaceae, or carrot, family, osha has for centuries been used medicinally by American Indians. It is an herbaceous perennial growing to more than 3 feet tall. It has lance-shaped leaves and white flowers that appear during the late summer. They are followed by small reddish fruits that are oblong in shape. The root is most often used as a remedy.

WHERE IT CAN BE FOUND:

Mexico, Montana, Wyoming, Colorado, New Mexico, California, Oregon, Arizona, Nevada, Utah

PROPERTIES AND USE:

Febrifuge, anti-inflammatory, antimicrobial, expectorant, antiviral, antivenomous, tonic, and treats respiratory infections, flu, rheumatism, sore throat, hangover, diarrhea, gastrointestinal conditions, wounds, skin conditions, heart conditions, sinus infections, altitude sickness, earache, catarrh, insect stings or bites, allergies, nicotine addiction.

TRADITIONAL PREPARATION:

For altitude sickness, chew the raw root. To make a decoction, boil 1 teaspoon chopped root in 1 cup water for 20 minutes. Steep for 20 minutes. Strain before drinking. This can also be used as a gargle, compress, rinse, or bath. It is available in tea, tincture, and vinegar forms. **To break a nicotine habit**, the hollow stems are smoked.

DID YOU KNOW?

Osha root has traditionally been used as a talisman.

Pejibaye

Like most palm trees, pejibaye grows tall, with one stem or a cluster of stems. It has black spines arranged in circular rows at its base and up the stem. The fruit is usually orange, yellow, or red in color when ripe. It grows to about the size of a plum, in clusters of up to hundreds of fruits. It has a texture similar to a sweet potato. The plant is usually harvested twice a year, in January and May. Common names include peach palm, *pixbae*, *pijuayo*, *pupunha*, and *peewah*.

WHERE IT CAN BE FOUND:

Native to the tropical forest areas in Central and South America, including Costa Rica, Honduras, Brazil, and Bolivia

PROPERTIES AND USE:

Anti-aging, hypotensive. Pejibaye is high in vitamins A and C, nicotinic acid, fat, and calories, making it a staple for many in Central and South America. Used to treat headache and stomachache.

TRADITIONAL PREPARATION:

Pejibaye is most commonly **used as a food**. Boil the fruit for 3 hours in salted water. Traditionally, pork fat is added to the water, but you can forego this. Drinking the salted water is used to treat headaches. You may also eat the young flowers on salad for headaches or stomachaches. **For headaches**, peel the fruit and mash it in a small bowl. Apply to the forehead. You may also use this as a facial mask.

DID YOU KNOW?

In some indigenous cultures, pejibaye was used as a dietary substitute for corn. Pejibaye was a better option, because it has higher nutritional content than corn. In addition, one average pejibaye fruit contains 1,096 calories, making it the perfect solution to malnutrition.

Peruvian Balsam

Growing to 60 feet tall, the Peruvian balsam's alternate, petioled leaves are odd-pinnate, with seven to 11 leaflets of 3 inches long. They're wide, rounded at the base, and pointed. The resin is brownish, with a bitter vanilla flavor and smoky odor. In addition to its medicinal uses, it is used widely in perfumes, soaps, and cosmetics.

WHERE IT CAN BE FOUND:

Central America, South America

PROPERTIES AND USE:

Antiparasitic, diuretic, alterative, expectorant, antifungal (especially for ringworm), and treats wounds, bruises, hemorrhoids, skin conditions, cavities and "dry socket", cancer, frostbite, burns

TRADITIONAL PREPARATION:

For skin conditions, burns, frostbite, and ringworm, apply the resin directly to the affected area. As an expectorant, combine 1 tablespoon resin with 1 large egg yolk. Drink. **As a treatment for cancer**, mix 1 tablespoon resin with 2 cups warm water. Sip throughout the day. **For hemorrhoids**, combine equal parts *Theobroma cacao* and Peruvian balsam resin, and apply directly to the affected area. It can also be made into a suppository by wrapping the mixture into plastic wrap, shaping it in the appropriate size, and chilling it for 1 hour. Remove from plastic and insert into the anus. **For cavities**, press the resin into the hole.

DID YOU KNOW?

Peruvian balsam is used in dental preparations used to treat "dry socket". It is also used in toothpaste and in some dental impression materials.

Pheasant Tail

This is a large herbaceous plant with dark green, leathery leaves and a dark purple bract on a tall spike. It bears small berries that are red when ripe.

WHERE IT CAN BE FOUND:

Mexico, Central America, Northern South America

PROPERTIES AND USE:

Antispasmodic, analgesic, and treats sprains, aches, rheumatism, arthritis, paralysis, backache, sore muscles, muscle spasms, inflammation, urinary tract infections

TRADITIONAL PREPARATION:

For all conditions, boil 3 large leaves in 2 gallons water for 10 minutes. **For severe conditions**, boil the leaves and place the affected area over the steam. Tent with a blanket, being careful not to burn yourself. **For pain and swelling**, make a poultice of mashes leaves. Wear throughout the day. **For urinary tract infections**, boil a handful of roots in 3 cups water for 10 minutes. Sip throughout the day. In Mexico, this decoction is given to **ease childbirth pains, and to facilitate healing after childbirth**.

DID YOU KNOW?

A recent clinical study showed that freeze-dried pheasant tail roots showed growth-inhibitory and apoptosis-inducing (programmed cell death) properties. Their findings showed "strong in vitro anticancer activity."

Physic Nut

Known as *piñon* in Honduras, physic nut is widely used in Maya medicine. It is a shrub that grows to more than 6 feet tall and has spreading branches with leaves that ooze a clear sap when broken from the stem. Its flowers are white.

WHERE IT CAN BE FOUND:

Caribbean, Africa, Australia, India, Middle East, Asia, Central America, Florida, Hawaii

PROPERTIES AND USE:

Treats arthritis, hot flashes, anger, backache, inflammation of the ovaries, vaginal conditions, mouth sores, infantile thrush, constipation, incontinence

TRADITIONAL PREPARATION:

For mouth sores, chew on and swallow a leaf and piece of stem at night. Repeat for three nights. **For infantile thrush**, rub the sap directly inside the mouth. For all conditions, boil 1 leaf per cup water. Consume 1 to 3 cups per day. **To treat**

arthritis, the roots of 9 young trees are chopped and soaked in 2 quarts water for one day; the infusion is sipped throughout the day.

Pineapple

With large leaves and a height of 3 feet or more, pineapples grow on a plant that is grounded with a thick stem. The surface of the fruit is scaly and irregularly shaped, with rough bark. Pineapple was named after the pinecone, because of its similar appearance. The flesh of the fruit is sweet and yellow, and very aromatic. Since 2000, most of the fresh pineapples sold in Europe and the United States are hybrid versions, which have lower acidity levels. Once a pineapple is harvested it will no longer ripen, so it is best to wait to harvest the fruit until after it has ripened.

WHERE IT CAN BE FOUND:

Caribbean, Central America, South America, Africa, the South Pacific, Philippines, Asia, Hawaii

PROPERTIES AND USE:

Anti-inflammatory, anti-aging, tonic, and used to treat cancer, digestion problems, sore throat, sinus infection, bruises, colds, poor immune system function, cancer, prostate conditions, sunspots, gout, arthritis, hay fever, obesity, colitis

TRADITIONAL PREPARATION:

It is best to eat pineapple fresh, because heat deactivates the enzymatic properties of bromelain. Cut off the top and the scaly bark, and the flesh of the fruit can be cut away from the hard-inner core and eaten. Another way to enjoy the medicinal benefits is by drinking fresh, unheated pineapple juice. In the Maya lands, going on a 10 to 30-day pineapple juice cleanse is said to **reduce the appearance of sunspots and detoxify the liver**.

DETOX SMOOTHIE
Makes 1 serving

This smoothie is so delicious, it's hard to believe it's medicinal.

INGREDIENTS:

- 2 slices pineapple, chopped

- 1/2 papaya, cubed

- 1/2 small apple, chopped

- 2 tablespoons plain yogurt

- Juice of 1/2 lemon

- 1 mint sprig

- Ground cinnamon, for garnish

INSTRUCTIONS:

- Blend all ingredients except the cinnamon

- Before serving, sprinkle with a bit of cinnamon which will add flavor and a boost of iron, calcium and manganese

Use:

Drink in place of breakfast

DID YOU KNOW?

If you cut off the top of a pineapple and plant it in the ground, a new pineapple plant will grow.

Pito

The pito tree grows tall and can reach heights of 30 to 40 feet. The flowers bloom red, and the pods are brownish in color. Inside the pods are red seeds. It is also known by the name of coral bean. This plant is easy to identify, but you need to be cautious while harvesting, since the leaves and uncooked beans are toxic.

WHERE IT CAN BE FOUND:

Caribbean, Central America

PROPERTIES AND USE:

Sedative, nervine, anti-hemorrhagic, and treats dysentery and a number of female conditions

TRADITIONAL PREPARATION:

To treat insomnia, tuck a flower in your pillow. **For stress, anxiety, and irritability**, add a small amount of flowers or beans to scrambled eggs, black or kidney beans, or meat. You may also prepare the young twigs, buds, and flowers as you would string beans. **For all conditions**, make a decoction of 1 tablespoon flowers in 1-gallon water. Bring to a boil. Strain, and sip 1 cup throughout the day or before bed.

DID YOU KNOW?

The leaves of the pito tree are unique because they are heliotropic. This means that they move throughout the day, changing their orientation to follow the sun's movement. This aids in photosynthesis.

Pleurisy Root

The pleurisy plant was named because of its successful treatment of pleurisy, or painful inflammation of the lungs and chest. It grows in clumps that are between 1 and 3 feet tall and has bright yellow-orange or orange flowers that grow in clusters. The stems are hairy, and the leaves are narrow. Even though pleurisy root is sometimes called milkweed, the stems do not produce milky sap like other types of milkweed. The medicinal properties of this plant can be gained through the root. Other common names include butterfly weed, swallow-wort, orange milkweed, colic root, wind root, and tuber root.

WHERE IT CAN BE FOUND:

Northern Mexico, Ontario, Quebec, and all US states except Washington, Oregon, Idaho, Nevada, North Dakota, Montana, Wyoming, Hawaii, and Alaska

PROPERTIES AND USE:

Anti-inflammatory, expectorant, antispasmodic, analgesic, febrifuge, and treats respiratory infections, cough, uterine conditions, flu (especially swine flu)

TRADITIONAL PREPARATION:

This plant is rarely encapsulated; it is usually available in teas and extracts. Traditionally, it was used by the indigenous American tribes who harvested it wild, and then dried the rhizome from the root and ground it up to make a topical paste. Pleurisy flowers, leaves, and young seedpods are edible, and they are best consumed cooked. It has been said that the pods taste similar to sweet peas. The roots of the plant can be harvested in the fall, and they can be dried to use in the future.

For all conditions, pour 1 cup boiling water over 1 teaspoon dried pleurisy root powder. Drink 3 cups per day.

DID YOU KNOW?

The nickname butterfly weed originated from the fact that the plant attracts a variety of butterflies, including the brightly colored monarchs.

Ponderosa Pine

All species of pine trees were once used as foods and medicines worldwide. This large conifer tree grows to 225 feet tall in the wild and lives as long as 600 years. It has dark yellow-green needles between 5 and 10 inches long that grow in bundles of three. The cones are oval and between 4 and 6 inches long. They grow upright but turn upside down at maturity to release the seed. The bark is dark brown to black. In maturity, it turns yellowish brown to reddish-orange and has irregularly furrowed, scaly plates.

WHERE IT CAN BE FOUND:

British Columbia, Western half of the US except for Kansas, and temperate regions of Europe

PROPERTIES AND USE:

Antibiotic, antibacterial, antiviral, diuretic, rubefacient, vermifuge, and treats bladder conditions, poor kidney function, respiratory conditions, wounds, acne, skin fungus

TRADITIONAL PREPARATION:

To make an infusion, pour 2 cups boiling water over a small handful of chopped fresh needles. Steep for 5 to 10 minutes, and then strain. **For wounds, acne, and skin fungus**, apply the sap directly to the affected area. **For respiratory conditions**, boil 2 teaspoons chopped fresh needles and 1 tablespoons sugar in 1/4 cup water until syrupy. Administer 2 teaspoons per day.

PINE VINEGAR
Makes 2 cups

This vinegar is popular in Scandinavia, where it is used for flavoring and as a natural antibiotic and vermifuge. You will need a 16-ounce jar with lid for this recipe. Any type of pine needle may be used.

INGREDIENTS:

- 1 1/4 cups fresh pine needles

- 2 cups apple cider vinegar

INSTRUCTIONS:

- Pack a jar three-quarters full of fresh pine needles. Pour in apple cider vinegar to fill the jar.

- Tightly screw on the lid, and place on a windowsill too steep for six weeks.

- After six weeks, store in a cool, dark area.

USE:

Take a tablespoon per day. This may be used as a rinse or bath for skin conditions.

DID YOU KNOW?

Native Americans ate pine needs, which are high in vitamin C, to ward off winter colds and flu.

Popcorn Flower

The popcorn flower, also known as *árbol del Hermano Pedro*, grows to 50 feet high, and has fleshly, elliptic leaves, white funnel-shaped flowers, and fleshy yellowish-green fruit.

WHERE IT CAN BE FOUND:

Parts of southern Mexico, El Salvador, Honduras, Panama, Guatemala

PROPERTIES AND USE:

Astringent, antifungal, digestive, analgesic, sedative, hypotensive, antidepressant, stops menstruation, and treats toothache, halitosis, heart disease

TRADITIONAL PREPARATION:

For all conditions, pour 1 cup boiling water over 2 teaspoons dried flowers. Drink warm. **For hair loss**, boil 1 cup dried flowers in 1-gallon water. Cool, and use as a rinse on clean hair.

DID YOU KNOW?

Ancient Maya used the flower and bark to flavor cacao. Due to the sweet fragrance, it was also used in ceremonies, as the gods were lured to the earth plane by sweet-smelling treats.

Pumpkin

The name "pumpkin" refers to several types of squash, and usually the traditional pumpkin, *Cucurbita pepo* L. It has orange, slightly ribbed yet smooth skin and a thick shell. The interior is filled with flesh and seeds. Pumpkin seeds are packed with magnesium, which is great for heart, bone, and teeth health. They also contain zinc, good for cell health, skin and eye health, and restful sleep.

WHERE IT CAN BE FOUND:

Caribbean, Mexico, Central America, Alabama, Arkansas, California, Connecticut, Georgia, Illinois, Kansas, Kentucky, Louisiana, Massachusetts, Michigan, Missouri, Mississippi, North Carolina, New Hampshire, New Mexico, Nevada, New York, Ohio, Pennsylvania, South Carolina, Tennessee, Texas, Utah, Virginia, West Virginia, Ontario, Quebec

PROPERTIES AND USE:

Anti-inflammatory, antifungal, antidepressant, antiparasitic, diuretic, and treats benign prostatic hyperplasia, kidney infections, bladder infections, headache, skin conditions, poor immune system function, high cholesterol, rheumatism, arthritis, sore muscles

TRADITIONAL PREPARATION:

To treat parasites and tapeworm, peel and crush 1/4 cup pumpkin seeds. Boil in 1-liter water for 30 minutes. Strain, and sip throughout the day for 5 days. **For skin conditions, headaches, rheumatism, arthritis, and sore muscles**, peel the skin from the pumpkin, and place it, cut side down, directly on the affected area. **For all other conditions**, eat at least 1/2 cup of pumpkin per day. It is great sautéed or served mashed like potatoes.

DID YOU KNOW?

The heaviest pumpkin, grown in Stillwater, Minnesota, weighed in over 1,810 pounds in 2010.

Quebracho Blanco

This hardwood tree has weeping branches, and yellow flowers that are hermaphrodite. They are a popular flavoring for food.

WHERE IT CAN BE FOUND:

Central America, Western and Southern South America

PROPERTIES AND USE:

Febrifuge, antimalarial, stimulant, tonic. Treats asthma and promotes dental health.

TRADITIONAL PREPARATION:

For dental health and as a natural tooth whitener, chew a small piece of bark each day. **For all conditions,** boil a 1-inch by 6-inch piece of bark in 1-gallon water. Steep for 30 minutes. Strain, and drink 1 cup per day.

Quebracho Negro

This hardwood legume tree can grow to 50 feet tall. Its canopy is rounded and dense. The fruit is a flat pod of 4 to 8 inches in length and containing numerous dark seeds. It is also known as false tamarind.

WHERE IT CAN BE FOUND:

Mexico, Central America

PROPERTIES AND USE:

Antiparasitic, astringent, and used for dental health

TRADITIONAL PREPARATION:

As an antiparasitic and astringent, boil a 1-inch by 4-inch piece of bark in 1-gallon water. Drink 1 glass before each meal. **For dental health**, chew the bark each day.

Rhodiola

This perennial flowering plant grows to more than a foot tall from a short, scaly rootstock. It is hardy and able to grow in frigid conditions. It was used by the Vikings, Chinese emperors, and the Greek physician Dioscorides. This variety grows reddish purple flowers. Other varieties grow yellow flowers.

WHERE IT CAN BE FOUND:

Scandinavia, Europe, Russia, Asia, Quebec, Newfoundland, Nunavut, Maine, Vermont, New York, Pennsylvania, Connecticut, North Carolina

PROPERTIES AND USE:

Antioxidant, adaptogen, antidepressant, stimulant, anti-aging, hepatoprotetive, aphrodisiac, and used to increase strength, mental capacity, and memory. It is also used to treat heart conditions, high cholesterol, cancer, tuberculosis, diabetes, colds, flu, impotence, deafness, poor immune system function, fatigue, altitude sickness

TRADITIONAL PREPARATION:

To make an infusion, boil 1 teaspoon chopped root in 1 cup water for 1 hour. Sip throughout the day.

RHODIOLA TINCTURE
Makes 3/4 cup

This is a popular tincture in Scandinavia, where Rhodiola is used to treat conditions including depression, fatigue, and memory loss. You can grind Rhodiola root in a coffee grinder, or purchase it ground. You will need an 8-ounce jar with lid for this recipe.

INGREDIENTS:

- 1-ounce ground Rhodiola root

- 3/4 cup 100-proof vodka

INSTRUCTIONS:

- Place the ground root in the jar. Pour in the vodka.

- Tightly screw on the lid and shake well. Allow too steep for 5 days at room temperature. Strain before use.

USE:

Take 1/2 teaspoon three times per day for 2 to 3 weeks.

DID YOU KNOW?

Athletes use Rhodiola to shorten the recovery time after workouts.

Rosemary

Rosemary is one of the most-lauded herbs we encountered along our travels throughout the Americas. We saw both Mediterranean rosemary (*Rosmarinus officinalis* L.) and Caribbean "rosemary" (*Croton linearis* – Jacq.). The former will likely be more widely available to you, no matter where you live. Though they are not in the same family, they do have similar healing properties. This woody, perennial herb has fragrant, evergreen, needle-like leaves and white, pink, purple, or blue flowers. Caribbean rosemary has longer leaves that are fewer in number.

WHERE IT CAN BE FOUND:

Western and Central Mediterranean, California, North Carolina, Oregon, South Carolina, Texas, cultivated elsewhere

PROPERTIES AND USE:

Tonic, astringent, digestive, carminative, hepatoprotective, antibacterial, diaphoretic, stomachic, nervine, rubefacient, abortifacient, hypotensive, emmenagogue, insecticidal, expectorant, and used for hair loss, skin conditions, dandruff, memory loss, Alzheimer's disease, headache, gout, cough, gallbladder conditions, anorexia, toothache, rheumatism, sore muscles, fibromyalgia, menstrual pain, PMS

TRADITIONAL PREPARATION:

For all conditions, place 1 cup fresh or 3 teaspoons dried rosemary in a small pot. Add 3 cups water. Bring to a boil. Continue boiling for 5 minutes. Remove from heat, and steep for 10 minutes. Drink as hot as you can. Cooled, this same decoction is **used to treat hair loss, dandruff, and to make hair shiny**. It is also used as a skin wash. **For congestion and coughs**, place a towel over the head, and inhale deeply as the decoction boils.

DID YOU KNOW?

Rosemary is used throughout the Caribbean to ward off negativity and malignant entities.

HERBAL HAIR INFUSION
Makes 6 treatments

This herbal hair rinse is great for removing build-up, flakes, and for making your hair shiny. It can also be used to prevent hair loss. It is not recommended for use on dry, damaged hair. You will need to prepare the infusion two hours before use. It is best used on brunettes, as the infusion can temporarily darken their hair, as well as towels with which it comes into contact. You will need a storage bottle for this recipe. An old shampoo bottle (washed, of course) works great.

INGREDIENTS:

- 2 cups distilled water

- 1/2 cup apple cider vinegar

- 2 tablespoons fresh chopped rosemary

- 2 tablespoons fresh chopped sage

- 1 tablespoon fresh chopped nettle

- 1 tablespoon fresh chopped lavender

- 5 drops tea tree essential oil

- 5 drops rosemary essential oil

INSTRUCTIONS:

- In a small saucepan, bring the water and vinegar to a simmer over medium heat. Remove from heat.

- Add the herbs, cover, and steep for 2 hours.

- Strain, and then stir in the essential oils.

- Carefully pour the infusion into your cleaned shampoo bottle. Refrigerate for up to 1 month.

USE:

Shake the bottle, and then apply approximately 1/4 cup of the infusion to washed or unwashed wet hair. Gently massage into the scalp and hair for 2 to 3 minutes, and then rinse.

Rue

The notion that a plant can provide protection is, perhaps, a bit strange in our modern thinking. And yet many plants—basil, rosemary, and tobacco among them—were once believed to possess profound spiritual abilities. Even today, people the world over believe in the energetic gifts of certain herbs. This hearty, evergreen shrub with yellow flowers is one of them. Derived from the Greek word rua, which means "to set free", rue is still believed by many to liberate people from disease, and energetically, from envy, evil eye, fear, and grief. Not surprisingly, it also possesses great medicinal benefits and is known as "herb of grace".

WHERE IT CAN BE FOUND:

Europe, Central America, South America, Alabama, California, Connecticut, District of Columbia, Illinois, Maryland, Missouri, North Carolina, New Jersey, New York, Pennsylvania, Rhode Island, Texas, Virginia, Vermont, Wisconsin, West Virginia, Alberta, Ontario, Quebec

PROPERTIES AND USE:

Stimulant, antispasmodic, emmenagogue, rubefacient, nervine, vermifuge, antivenomous, carminative, and treats stomach cramps, epilepsy, vomiting, difficult childbirth, rheumatism, sore muscles, headache, backache, exhaustion, cough, multiple sclerosis, sciatica

TRADITIONAL PREPARATION:

For all conditions, squeeze the extract of 9 small, leafy branches into a glass of lukewarm water. Strain, and drink twice daily before meals. Pregnant women begin sipping it once contractions begin, and then throughout labor. Pregnant women should not use rue until labor. **For rheumatism, headaches, and backaches**, soak rue leaves in alcohol, and place on the affected area. You can also use the alcohol-soaked leaves to massage sore muscles, or those suffering from fever or exhaustion. **For coughs**, boil 1 leaf in 1/4 cup water and 1 teaspoon sugar until it is syrupy. Administer by the teaspoon as necessary. **For spiritual disease, such as envy, evil eye, fear, and grief**, place sprigs in a cross formation over your doorway so that all who enter your house are cleansed. If you have recently been the target of **negativity or envy**, place a small sprig under your tongue until it dissolves. For snakebites, mash the leaves and pack into the fang marks. **For sciatica**, bruise the leaves and place directly on the affected area.

RUE SALVE

Makes about 3 cups

To make this recipe, you will need either a slow cooker or double boiler, which you can fashion yourself with a metal mixing bowl and slightly smaller pot filled with a bit of water. Rue Salve is excellent for massaging areas affected by rheumatism, sore muscles, fibromyalgia, sciatica, carpal tunnel syndrome, or other conditions.

INGREDIENTS:

- 2 cups olive oil

- 1/3 cup chopped rue leaves

- 1-liter water

- 2/3 cup beeswax

INSTRUCTIONS:

- Place the first three ingredients in your slow cooker or double boiler. Simmer for 4 hours, stirring from time to time.

- Remove from heat and allow to cool enough to handle. Strain through a fine-mesh sieve, pressing the rue with the back of a spoon to extract all the oils. Discard the rue.

- Chill for 24 to 48 hours, until the water and oil separate. Skim off the water, and discard.

- Place the oil in a heavy saucepan and simmer over low heat. Do not allow to come to a boil.

- Add the beeswax, stirring until dissolved.

- Pour into storage containers with lids.

USE:

Massage directly onto the affected area

Sanchezia

Sanchezia is a bushy shrub with sturdy, bright green or purple stems and large, green leaves with light-green veins. Its tubular yellow, orange, and red flowers grow in spikes.

WHERE IT CAN BE FOUND:

Caribbean, Central America, South America, South Pacific

PROPERTIES AND USE:

Antitumor, nervine, tonic, and treats heart conditions, sore muscles, arthritis, rheumatism, painful menstruation

TRADITIONAL PREPARATION:

To make a decoction, boil a handful of leaves in 1-gallon water for 30 minutes. Remove from heat, and then steep for 30 minutes. Drink 1 cup per day. You may also juice the leaves and drink up to 1/2 cup per day.

Sangre De Grado

This medium- to large-sized tree grows to 65 feet tall in the upper Amazon. The trunk is covered by smooth, mottled bark. Its large green leaves are heart shaped, and its light green or white flowers grow on large stalks. Its name translates to "dragon's blood", so named because when the trunk is wounded or cut, it oozes a dark red sap resembling blood.

WHERE IT CAN BE FOUND:

Peruvian Amazon, Mexico, Central America, Dominican Republic, Brazil

PROPERTIES AND USE:

Astringent, anesthetic, antibacterial, antiseptic, antitumor, antiviral, antihemorrhagic, antifungal, blood tonic, purgative, tonic. Used to treat wounds, fractures, vaginal and uterine conditions, infertility, rheumatism, intestinal conditions, insect bites, mouth sores, tonsillitis, sore throat, herpes, hemorrhoids, vaginal discharge, diarrhea, dysentery, colitis, and peptic ulcers.

TRADITIONAL PREPARATION:

For fractures, apply the bark as a poultice. **For wounds, skin conditions, insect bites, and fungus**, apply the sap directly to the affected area. **For all other conditions**, ingest the undiluted resin. It is recommended to not consume more than 2 tablespoons per day.

DID YOU KNOW?

In Europe and the US, sangre de grado resin is prescribed for nerve pain and inflammation.

Santa Maria

This large, green-leafed plant is also called monkey's hand due to its finger-like fruit spikes. These fruits are important to bat and bird species in its native Central America.

WHERE IT CAN BE FOUND:

Southeast Asia, South Pacific Islands, Africa, Mexico, Central America, South America, Caribbean, Florida

PROPERTIES AND USE:

Antispasmodic, antimalarial, anti-inflammatory, antibacterial, analgesic, antioxidant, anti-aging, febrifuge, antiparasitic, and used to treat kidney infections, diarrhea, skin conditions, burns, rheumatism, earache, poor lactation

TRADITIONAL PREPARATION:

For skin conditions and burns, apply the juice from the leaves directly to the skin. You may also wrap the affected area with a leaf. **For earaches**, squeeze the juice from the leaves directly into the ear. **For all other conditions**, boil a handful of roots and leaves in 1-gallon water for 30 minutes. Steep at least an hour or overnight, and then strain. Drink up to 1 cup per day.

DID YOU KNOW?

Santa maria leaves are used as plates, tablecloths, and wrappers for food and other items.

Santo Domingo

Also known as Aztec tobacco, *mapacho tobacco*, or rome, santo domingo is a plant used widely in shamanic ritual.

Considered by various American tribes to be one of the oldest, most powerful plants on the planet, it is said to cleanse one's life of negative energies. It is often used with ayahuasca. Santo domingo has a higher nicotine content than cultivated tobacco. Its flowers are bright greenish-yellow.

WHERE IT CAN BE FOUND:

Mexico, Central America, South America, Africa, India, Russia, Scandinavia, South Australia, Connecticut, Illinois, Massachusetts, Michigan, Minnesota, Missouri, North Carolina, New Hampshire, New Jersey, New Mexico, New York, Ohio, Oregon, Pennsylvania, South Carolina, Virginia, Wisconsin, Ontario

PROPERTIES AND USE:

Antivenomous, antiseptic, antifungal, carminative, digestive, nervine, vermifuge, antispasmodic, antimalarial. Used to treat acid reflux, hemorrhoids, nasal polyps, hernia, constipation, epilepsy, respiratory infections, lice, wounds, hair loss, earache, negativity.

TRADITIONAL PREPARATION:

For all conditions, it is smoked by a shaman or healer, who rolls dried leaves into a cigarette and blows the smoke on the affected area. **For hernias, acid reflux, nasal polyps, anxiety, gas, and epileps**y, dried leaves can be rolled and smoked like a cigarette. **For snakebites**, it is chewed and then packed into the fang marks. This may also be done with fungus or wounds. **For constipation or epilepsy**, boil 3 dried leaves in 1-gallon water. Drink 1/2 cup as needed. Cooled, this decoction can be used as a nasal rinse for nasal polyps, and as a rinse for hair loss. **For earache**, roll a dried leaf and place directly into the ear.

DID YOU KNOW?

Native peoples scatter santo domingo to the ground as an offering to Creator. It is often done in four directions while praying. Because of its protective properties, it is scattered outside a home, and in corners within a house.

Saw Palmetto

As a small palm, saw palmetto only reaches a maximum height of 6 feet. It grows with a sprawling trunk, or in dense clumps along sandy coastal areas. This plant lives for a long time and is very slow growing. The leaves look like a fan, with about 20 leaflets each. These leaves have small spines or teeth that can cut the skin, so be cautious and use gloves when touching the plant. Its flowers are yellowish-white in color, and its fruit is reddish-black. Most of the medicinal benefits are gained from its fruit. Other common names include palmetto, dwarf palm tree, and sabal serrulatum.

WHERE IT CAN BE FOUND:

Alabama, Florida, Georgia, Louisiana, Mississippi, South Carolina, Texas

PROPERTIES AND USE:

Anti-inflammatory, diuretic, expectorant, digestive, nervine, aphrodisiac, antiseptic, tonic. Treats reproductive conditions in men and women. Soothes the digestive tract, boosts appetite, and increases nutrient assimilation. Heals benign prostatic hyperplasia and respiratory conditions including chronic cough, bronchitis, asthma, laryngitis, and whooping cough.

TRADITIONAL PREPARATION:

For all conditions, boil 1 tablespoon dried saw palmetto berries, 1 teaspoon maca powder, and 1/2 teaspoon cinnamon in 1 cup water for 10 minutes. Optionally, you may wish to add ginger and honey. Strain, and drink warm. For reproductive and bladder problems, eat the fruit. For energy, juice the fruit, and consume 2 ounces per day before breakfast.

Scorpion Tail

Because of its beauty, many people use scorpion tail as a decorative plant, not realizing it offers medicinal benefits, as well. It is an upright herb growing to about 3 feet tall. It has rough, green leaves and small, white flowers that grow on a curled stem. A relative, *Heliotropium angiospermum*, grows in Florida and Texas and possesses similar medicinal properties.

WHERE IT CAN BE FOUND:

Tropical Asia, Africa, Caribbean, Central America, Mexico, South America, Alabama, Arkansas, Florida, Georgia, Illinois, Indiana, Kansas, Kentucky, Louisiana, Massachusetts, Maryland, Missouri, Mississippi, North Carolina, New York, Ohio, Oklahoma, South Carolina, Tennessee, Texas, Virginia, West Virginia

PROPERTIES AND USE:

Astringent, emollient, diuretic, febrifuge, aphrodisiac, emmenagogue, and treats skin conditions, wounds, diarrhea, conjunctivitis, painful menstruation, infant malaise and vomiting

TRADITIONAL PREPARATION:

For painful menstruation, boil a small handful of stem pieces in 3 cups water for 5 minutes. Do not exceed 3 cups per day or continue for more than a few days, as it can be toxic. **For all conditions**, boil 3 leaves in 1 cup water for 10 minutes. Strain before drinking. Cooled, it can be used as an eyewash. **For infant diarrhea, malaise, and vomiting**, boil an entire scorpion tail in 1-gallon water for 5 minutes. Bathe the child in the warm water before bed. **For skin conditions or wounds**, macerate the leaves and apply as a poultice.

Sea Almond Tree

The sea almond tree originated in the East Indies but has become a popular natural remedy around the world. Sea almond trees grow tall and can reach heights between 50 and 100 feet. The crown of the tree is upright and symmetrical, with branches that grow horizontally and tiered. Leaves on the sea almond tree are green and large, with a glossy and leathery texture. The seedpods of this plant are similar in appearance to large, unshelled almonds. They are about 3 inches in length, and the outside of the pod is inedible. The seeds, like the fruit, can be used internally or topically. Other names for this tree include Bengal almond, country almond, tropical almond, Malabar almond, and Indian almond. On the Caribbean island of Roatán it is called hammond leaf.

WHERE IT CAN BE FOUND:

Central America, Caribbean, India, Asia, Africa, Brazil, Australia, Peru, Florida, Hawaii

PROPERTIES AND USE:

Febrifuge, hypotensive. Treats rheumatism, eye problems, headaches, mouth and throat problems, asthma, cough, colic.

Beneficial for wounds and skin conditions. Soothes digestive problems such as diarrhea, stomachache, motion sickness, and dysentery. Stops bleeding from an extracted tooth.

TRADITIONAL PREPARATION:

For all conditions, consume 1/2 cup leaf, fruit, and seed juice per day. The juice can also be applied topically **to soothe skin conditions and to cleanse wounds**. In addition, for all conditions, the fruit can be eaten raw, or its seed oil can be extracted for consumption. **For wounds, skin conditions, and rheumatism**, soak a 1-inch by 9-inch piece of bark in water overnight. Break the soaked bark apart and use it as a poultice. The liquid can be drunk **for diarrhea, dysentery, and fever. To stop bleeding** from an extracted tooth, pack with chewed leaves.

DID YOU KNOW?

Despite its name, this plant is not related to the almonds that are common in grocery stores.

Sea Grape

True to its name, this plant grows near the ocean, and its fruit resembles small clusters of grapes. When the fruit begins to grow in the late summer, it is a greenish color, eventually ripening to purple when it is ready to harvest. The leaves of this small tree are large and broad and look like a fan. Other common names include bay grape, shore-grape, platterleaf, and tagalog.

WHERE IT CAN BE FOUND:

Caribbean, Central America, Colombia, Ecuador, Florida, Hawaii, Mississippi

PROPERTIES AND USE:

Antibacterial, antifungal, astringent, hypoglycemic, anti-inflammatory, and treats nausea, diarrhea, mouth sores, sore throat, gum disease, asthma, cancer

TRADITIONAL PREPARATION:

The bark of the sea grape tree was traditionally boiled and used as a remedy **for diarrhea**. The young leaves can be boiled, and the infused water used as a mouthwash and gargle to treat **oral infections**. To prepare an extract, the leaves can be boiled for 4 hours to draw out the compounds. The fruit is edible, and often made into jellies, jams, or wine. The flowers produce nectar, and good quality honey. **To treat fungus**, macerate the leaves and apply directly to the affected area.

DID YOU KNOW?

Before modern-day candies were available, children used to eat sea grapes as a sweet treat.

Senna

A small shrub with green leaves, orange-yellow flowers, and pods containing up to eight seeds, Senna is a popular laxative. This natural remedy should be used with caution, however, because long-term use could potentially lead to organ failure.

WHERE IT CAN BE FOUND:

Africa, India, Caribbean, Mexico, Mediterranean

PROPERTIES AND USE:

Laxative, and therefore sometimes used for weight loss

TRADITIONAL PREPARATION:

Pour 1 cup boiling water over 1/4 teaspoon dried Senna leaves. Steep for 10 minutes, strain, and then drink warm. **For severe constipation**, add 1 small pod to the infusion.

Soursop

The soursop tree is a flowering evergreen with broad leaves. It produces a fruit often touted as a natural remedy for cancer, as well as for other medical conditions. The shape of the fruit varies and can grow to the size of a watermelon. It is dark green in the beginning, and then lightens into a yellowish-green color when ripe. The skin is spiny send leathery, and the flesh soft when ripe.

WHERE IT CAN BE FOUND:

Caribbean, Central America, Southeast Asia, and other topical areas worldwide

PROPERTIES AND USE:

Anti-inflammatory, antitumor, hypoglycemic, sedative, antibacterial, nervine, antiparasitic, hypotensive, antiviral, antispasmodic, digestive, vermifuge, febrifuge, emetic (in large doses), insecticidal. Used to boost endocrine and thyroid activity. It is also used for cancer, and conditions of the bladder, pancreas, and kidneys.

TRADITIONAL PREPARATION:

For all conditions, peel and eat the fruit. One-half cup per day is recommended. **To make an infusion**, pour boiling water over 1 leaf. Steep for 10 minutes, and then drink warm. Drink 3 cups per day. The standard dosage for capsules or tablets is 2 grams three times per day.

DID YOU KNOW?

Even though the taste of the soursop fruit is sour, there is a hint of sweet that is described as being similar to a mix between a pineapple and strawberry. Its texture is creamy, similar to banana.

Squash Seed

Cucurbita ficifolia is a perennial, climbing vine that grows to 45 feet in length. Its fruit is oblong and resembles a watermelon. Its flowers are yellow to orange. Other common names include the seven-year melon and the fig leaf gourd.

WHERE IT CAN BE FOUND:

Mexico to Chile, Africa highlands, India, Asia, Philippines, California

PROPERTIES AND USE:

Hypoglycemic, anti-inflammatory, antiaging, vermifuge, detoxifying, and treats sore muscles and diabetes

TRADITIONAL PREPARATION:

To detoxify, mix 1 teaspoon ground squash seed or 1/2 teaspoon squash seed extract with the juice of 1/2 lemon in 12 ounces room temperature water. This is especially powerful when fasting or on a cleanse. **To make a decoction**, boil 2 tablespoons squash seeds in 3 cups water for 30 minutes. Drink before meals.

DID YOU KNOW?

Squash seed extract is effectively used to treat pre-diabetes and type 2 diabetes. It is not yet known if it is effective for treating type 1 diabetes.

St. John's Wort

St. John's wort is renowned for its treatment of depression, but it possesses other medicinal benefits, as well. It is an erect, multi-stemmed, perennial forb that grow to 3 feet tall. It has long, slender "runners" growing on and just below the soil surface. Its numerous flowers are symmetrical around a central point, growing in flat-topped clusters. They are bright yellow-orange and edged with black dots. Other common names include Klamath weed, chase-devil, goat weed, rosin rose, and Tipton's weed.

WHERE IT CAN BE FOUND:

Europe, Africa, Asia, Northern Africa, Middle East, all US states except Alabama, Arizona, Florida, Utah

PROPERTIES AND USE:

Antidepressant, antibacterial, antifungal, nervine. Used for heart palpitations, anxiety, exhaustion, fibromyalgia, chronic fatigue syndrome, seasonal affective disorder, smoking cessation, sore muscles, nerve pain, irritable bowel syndrome, skin conditions, PMS, hepatitis C, migraine, headache, obsessive-compulsive disorder, ADHD, symptoms of menopause, hemorrhoids, burns, wounds

TRADITIONAL PREPARATION:

St. John's wort can be purchased in tea, pill, or liquid form. A common dosage is 2 to 4 grams three times per day. **For all conditions**, pour 1 cup boiling water over 1 to 2 teaspoons dried leaves. Steep for 5 minutes. Strain and drink in one sitting. Cooled, this can be used as a rinse or bath for **skin conditions, burns, and wounds**.

DID YOU KNOW?

St. John's wort gained its name from St. John the Baptist, as the plant blooms around the time of his feast (June 24). The name Hypericum comes from the Greek language: hyper, meaning above, and eikon, meaning picture. It references the ancient tradition of hanging the plant over a religious icon. This was believed to ward off evil.

Strongback

Strongback is the Maya world's most powerful medicine for adult asthma. It is also, true to its name, excellent at treating backache. It is a weedy, perennial herb that grows to 1 ½ feet tall and has numerous lavender-colored flowers. The green fruits grow in beanlike pods.

Three other plants, *Morinda royac, Desmodium canum*, and *Cuphea parsonsia* are also called strongback. All four have similar properties.

WHERE IT CAN BE FOUND:

Mexico, Caribbean, Central America, Amazon, tropical Asia, West Coast of Africa

PROPERTIES AND USE:

Antispasmodic, nervine, analgesic, antifungal, anti-inflammatory, detoxifier, diuretic, mildly laxative, anti-allergen, and used to treat wounds, asthma, backache, allergies, water retention

TRADITIONAL PREPARATION:

For asthma, muscle spasms, and constipation, mash fresh leaves (the younger the better) with a bit of salt. Administer three times per day. **For backaches, allergies, and water retention**, pour 1 cup boiling water over 3 leaves. Drink warm. Repeat up to twice per day. **For fungus and wounds**, mash or chew the leaves and place directly on the affected area. For bad wounds, roast the roots, and crush into a powder. Apply directly to the wound.

DID YOU KNOW?

Capsules sold as "Desmodium" are strongback.

Sweetsop

Before the colonization of the Americas, sweetsop was an important foodstuff and medicine to indigenous tribes. It is a medium-sized shrub, with purple-flecked, jade-colored flowers that grow in clusters. The mature fruit has a purple or black coloring when ripe, and it is covered in leathery scales. When the outer skin is removed, the flesh has a gooey consistency and sweet smell and taste. Other common names include custard apple, sugar apple, bull's heart, and bullock's heart.

WHERE IT CAN BE FOUND:

Tropical Central America, tropical South America, Southern Mexico, Caribbean, Asia, Australia, Philippines, Florida

PROPERTIES AND USE:

Antibacterial, anti-inflammatory, antiparasitic, hypotensive, emollient, and treats skin conditions, burns, lice, arthritis, sore muscles, rheumatism, gout, indigestion, diarrhea, painful menstruation, colic

TRADITIONAL PREPARATION:

Sweetsop fruit can be eaten raw and is often added to desserts, jellies, and jams. **For skin conditions and burns,** make a poultice with the unripened fruit's flesh. It can also be used as a facial mask and **to soothe skin irritations and**

acne. Sweetsop leaves can be brewed or used as a decoction **to help with digestive problems**. Philippine shamans use the bark and roots to make a tonic **to help with colic, indigestion, and diarrhea**.

Tapaculo

Whether it's called bay cedar, *mutamba, pixoy, embira, baysi, cablote*, or any of its many other names, *Guazuma ulmifolia* is revered for its diarrhea-stopping abilities. It's also great for skin conditions and prostate problems.

Tapaculo is a large shrub growing to 100 feet tall, with grey-brown bark and a rounded crown. The leaves are 2 to 6 inches long, with serrated edges. Its small flowers are white to greenish-yellow, grow in clusters, and are quite fragrant. The fruit is woody and globose to broadly oval and 3/4 of an inch to 1 1/2 inches long. It is and black and covered with barbs when ripe.

WHERE IT CAN BE FOUND:

Caribbean, Central America, South America, Mexico, India, Indonesia, Netherlands, Panama

PROPERTIES AND USE:

Febrifuge, nervine, antibacterial, antifungal, digestive, hepatoprotective, antitumor, detoxifier, hypotensive, and is used for diarrhea, dysentery, asthma, cough, colds, intestinal issues, postpartum inflammation, sores, prostate conditions, rheumatism, bleeding, ulcers, skin conditions, difficult childbirth

TRADITIONAL PREPARATION:

For diarrhea and dysentery, crush three 1-inch by 3-inch pieces of bark. Boil in 1-liter water. Drink 1/4 cup every four hours as needed. **For cancer**, boil 2 handfuls of bark and boil in 1-gallon water. Remove from heat, and steep overnight. Drink 3 cups per day. For inflammation, boil three fruits in 2 cups water. Strain before drinking. **For skin conditions**, boil a large handful of chopped bark in 1-gallon water boil for 10 minutes. Allow to cool. Bathe the affected area three times per day and allow to air dry. **For dysentery and diarrhea**, boil a small handful bark in 3 cups water for 10 minutes. Sip throughout the day. Adding a touch of honey makes it a treatment **for prostate conditions and to aid difficult childbirth**.

DID YOU KNOW?

While traveling, it might not always be practical to make your own decoction. But you also might want to shy away from over-the-counter medications. Simply eat a few fresh tapaculo fruits, including the barbed outer layer, and you'll feel better in no time. You can find tapaculo in pastures, fields, and forests.

Thyme

Thyme has for centuries been used as a culinary herb, ornamental plant, and medicinal. The stems are wiry and narrow, with evergreen leaves and dense purple, white, or yellow flowers. Highly fragrant, it can repel beetles and other garden pests.

WHERE IT CAN BE FOUND:

Southern Europe, Mediterranean, Delaware, Massachusetts, New York, Pennsylvania, and cultivated elsewhere

PROPERTIES AND USE:

Antibacterial, anti-inflammatory, antispasmodic, expectorant, carminative, and treats cancer, cold, bronchitis, whooping cough, earache, swollen tonsils, nausea, diarrhea, gum disease, sore throat. Boosts immunity and improves concentration.

TRADITIONAL PREPARATION:

For all conditions, pour 1/2 cup boiling water over 1 teaspoon dried leaves. Steep for 10 minutes. **For coughs**, repeat up to 3 times per day. **For gum disease, swollen tonsils, sore throat**, rinse the mouth and make a gargle with thyme essential oil and water.

DID YOU KNOW?

In ancient times, thyme was used as incense. It comes from the Greek word for "to fumigate".

Tobacco

Tobacco has been referred to as "the intelligent herb", because it seems to do whatever is needed in the body to promote healing. The principle alkaloid is lobeline, which is similar to nicotine in chemical structure, but has the opposite effect: it relaxes muscles and decreases blood pressure. Tobacco can grow as tall as 3 feet, and it has a fragile flower that ranges in color from blue to violet, with a hint of yellow. Other common names include puke weed, bladder pod, Indian tobacco, asthma weed, and gagroot.

WHERE IT CAN BE FOUND:

Eastern North America from Southeastern Canada through the Eastern US to Alabama, and west to Kansas

PROPERTIES AND USE:

Hypotensive, antispasmodic, emetic (in large doses), and reduces nausea, muscle pain, and heart rate. It is used to treat PMS, poor digestion, whooping cough, respiratory infections, bronchitis, poor lymphatic flow, asthma

TRADITIONAL PREPARATION:

The parts above ground can be used for medicinal purposes, and generally the root is not used. The seeds are the most potent part of the plant. Tobacco is considered a "toxic" herb, and so it is best to start with smaller doses and increase the dosage as needed. It can be found in various forms, including extract, tincture, capsules, or as a dried herb. When using the dried herb, pour 1 cup boiling water over 1 teaspoon dried leaves. Steep for 10 minutes, and strain before drinking.

DID YOU KNOW?

The self-taught American herbalist and botanist Samuel Thomson is credited for discovering the medicinal uses of this herb. Legend holds that chewing on the leaves made him vomit, and so he gave it to his friends a "gag" ...hence the common name gagroot.

Topa

This frequently buttressed tree grows to 100 feet and has very large, heartshaped leaves. It has a spreading crown and grey or brown bark. The inner bark is yellowish, creamy white, or pinkish in color, turning brown with age. It has a single flower at the terminal end of the branch. The light heartwood was historically used for rafts. It is also known as *polak, algodón, palo de balsa, tambor*, corkwood, and *urú*.

WHERE IT CAN BE FOUND:

Southern Mexico to Bolivia, Caribbean

PROPERTIES AND USE:

Antitumor, analgesic, emetic, and used to treat osteoporosis, rheumatism, tuberculosis

TRADITIONAL PREPARATION:

A decoction of the leaves is drunk and used as a bath.

Trumpet Tree

Also known as *yarumo, yagrumo, embauba,* Cecropia, or *guarumo,* trumpet tree is a deciduous tree with a narrow trunk, and large, circular, leaves that are lobed. The flowers are pinkish-white succulent spikes that grow in clusters.

WHERE IT CAN BE FOUND:

The Andes, Caribbean, Central America, Northern South America, Africa, Asia, the Pacific

PROPERTIES AND USE:

Anti-inflammatory, hypotensive, sedative, antispasmodic, hepatoprotective, antihemorrhagic, febrifuge, cholagogue, analgesic, astringent, aphrodisiac, antibacterial, antifungal, hypoglycemic, emmenagogue. Treats asthma, broken bones,

STDs, Parkinson's disease, diabetes, ADHD, Tourette's syndrome, multiple sclerosis, Alzheimer's disease, Huntington's disease, migraine, sore throat, rheumatism, sore muscles, kidney conditions. Induces labor. Helps reduce weight.

TRADITIONAL PREPARATION:

For all conditions, steep 1 leaf in 2 cups water for 20 minutes. Consume 1 cup twice daily for three days. This same infusion is used as a gargle **for sore throats. For fevers**, boil 2 leaves in 1-quart water for 5 minutes. Place the leaves on the forehead and sip the decoction. Cooled, this can also be used as a soak or compress for rheumatism or broken bones. Also, **for rheumatism and for sore muscles**, you may tie a bundle of leaves and hang over your showerhead so that the water runs over the leaves. Shower in hot water, so that the leaves create an aromatic steam bath effect. This can also be done in the bath. **For stress**, smoke the dried leaves as a cigarette.

Turmeric

Turmeric is a flower plant of the ginger family. The plant is perennial plant native to India and southeast Asia. Plants are gathered each year for their roots, some for propagation in the following season and some for consumption.

WHERE IT CAN BE FOUND:

Native to India and Southeast Asia.

PROPERTIES AND USE:

It is used for many health conditions, including weight loss, lowering high cholesterol, burning fat more efficiently, and aiding in digestion. It is said to be good for the liver and kidneys. It is also used as a compress or wash to soothe the skin. Many arthritis patients use it for pain relief because of its anti-inflammatory properties and claim it works just as well as over the counter or even prescription medicines, but with fewer risks of side effects.

TRADITIONAL PREPARATION:

Can be taken in capsule form, it can also be used with nut milk or coconut milk. Some people make it into "Golden Milk," a type of turmeric tea with other spices, including turmeric, cinnamon, ginger and pepper.

Ubos

Also known as hog plum, ubos is a stately and erect tree with many medicinal properties. It has a corky bark, a buttressed trunk, with large leaves that are hairy underneath. The flowers are small and fragrant, and the fruits are similar to a plum. The ubos fruits grow in clusters, and they are a golden-yellow color when ripe. The skin of the fruit is tough, and the pulp is very juicy and acidic.

WHERE IT CAN BE FOUND:

Caribbean, Mexico, Central America, South America

PROPERTIES AND USE:

Abortifacient, antibacterial, antitumor, antiseptic, antispasmodic, nervine, antiviral, anti-inflammatory, sedative, diuretic, hypotensive, astringent, vermifuge, stomachic, tonic, analgesic, laxative, febrifuge. Treats candida and other vaginal infections, poor lactation, colic, diarrhea, sore throat, cough, herpes, gonorrhea, skin conditions, insect bites, headache. Induces labor, controls bleeding after childbirth, and is used as a contraceptive.

TRADITIONAL PREPARATION:

For diarrhea, gonorrhea, and sore throat, boil a handful of ubos buds and bark in 3 cups water for 10 minutes.

Drink a cup before meals. Continue for 10 days when treating gonorrhea. **For skin conditions, insect bites, and weakness during the second or third trimester of pregnancy**, boil 2 large handfuls of leaves and a 1-inch by 6-inch strip of bark in 2 gallons water for 10 minutes. Use as a bath. You may also rub bruised leaves directly on the affected area. **For fever and headaches**, macerate the leaves in a bit of alcohol, and apply directly on the head overnight for up to three nights. **For all conditions**, boil 3 cups water. Add 9 dried and crushed leaves, and a 3-inch piece of stem. Continue boiling, uncovered, for 30 minutes. Strain before drinking. Drink 3 cups per day.

Valerian

Valerian is a perennial flowering plant native to Europe and Asia. It will grow to 5 ft. tall during the summer growing season.

WHERE IT CAN BE FOUND:

Valerian is native to Europe and Asia. It is now being grown in North America.

PROPERTIES AND USE:

Valerian is commonly prescribed as a sedative and sleep aid that can relieve anxiety and help with insomnia.

It is also used for pain relief and chronic fatigue. Some people also use it to relieve the hyperactivity in Attention Deficit-Hyperactivity Disorder (ADHD).

TRADITIONAL PREPARATION:

Valerian products are available in capsule form. The valerian root can be used to make a tea.

Venadillo

The wood of the venadillo tree is used to construct furniture, and because of this, has become overexploited in some areas. The tree is small to medium in size, and grows a pear-shaped fruit containing many winged seeds. The fruit seems to defy gravity, because it grows upwards, earning it the name sky fruit. Other common names include *zapaton, gateago, cobano,* and Pacific mahogany.

WHERE IT CAN BE FOUND:

Mexico, Central America, Caribbean

PROPERTIES AND USE:

Hypotensive, hypoglycemic, antimalarial, anti-inflammatory, antibacterial, and treatshepatitis C, diarrhea, erectile dysfunction, skin conditions, sore muscles, cough, cancer, chest pain, stomachache

TRADITIONAL PREPARATION:

For all conditions, boil 1 tablespoon venadillo seeds in 1 cup water. Strain before drinking.

Verbena

Originally native to Europe, this perennial grows to 2 feet tall and has lobed leaves. Its mauve flowers grow from delicate spikes. It is known as holy herb, herb of the cross, wild hyssop, and mosquito plant. Another of its names, vervain, comes from the Celtic word *ferfaen—fer*, meaning to drive away and *faen*, meaning stone. Not surprisingly, it was used to treat bladder stones. It was also used to drive away malignant energies.

WHERE IT CAN BE FOUND:

Europe, Africa, Australia, Mexico, Central America, South America, California, New Mexico, Colorado, Wisconsin, Michigan, Oregon, Washington, New York, Pennsylvania, Massachusetts, Rhode Island, Connecticut, Delaware, New Jersey, District of Columbia, Virginia, North Carolina, South Carolina, Florida, Georgia, West Virginia, Kentucky, Tennessee, Arkansas, Mississippi, Louisiana

PROPERTIES AND USE:

Analgesic, antibacterial, antispasmodic, antitumor, astringent, diaphoretic, antidepressant, tonic, stimulant, emmenagogue, nervine, febrifuge. Used to treat rheumatism, poor lactation, wounds, itching, eczema, gall bladder conditions, exhaustion, minor injuries, gum disease, symptoms of menopause, painful menstruation, stomach conditions, liver conditions, spleen conditions, urinary tract infections, bladder stones

TRADITIONAL PREPARATION:

For all conditions, pour 1 cup boiling water over 1 teaspoon dried Verbena leaves and flowers. Steep for 5 minutes, and then strain. Repeat up to two times per day. This may be used as a wash **for itching and eczema**, and as a gargle **for gum disease**. Alternatively, take one to three tablespoons Verbena tincture, often sold as vervain extract, each day.

DID YOU KNOW?

You've seen that many of the herbs contained in this guide have a scientific name containing *officinalis*. This is because it's Latin for "used in medicine or herbalism".

Wax Jambu

The wax jambu tree grows to 50 feet tall, and when mature, can bear up to 2,000 fruits per year. The fruit is bell shaped, with waxy skin and a sweet-sour taste. Because the fruit can have different colors, it is best to determine the ripeness based on the texture. It should be fi rm to the touch, and crisp to the bite. In addition to the fruit, the bark and roots possess medicinal properties. Other common names include rose apple, water apple, bell fruit, and love apple.

WHERE IT CAN BE FOUND:

Fiji, India, Indonesia, Malaysia, Central America, and other tropical areas worldwide

PROPERTIES AND USE:

Diuretic, hypotensive, expectorant, hepatoprotective, febrifuge, and treats diabetes, Alzheimer's disease, diarrhea, digestive conditions, cancer (particularly breast and prostate), poor brain function, cold, flu, sore throat, coronary heart disease, high cholesterol, pancreas conditions, skin conditions, rheumatism

TRADITIONAL PREPARATION:

For all conditions, eating the fruit is recommended. You can also make a tea by boiling 1 whole fruit in 1-liter water. Strain, and sip throughout the day. **For skin conditions and rheumatism**, powder the dried leaves, and apply directly to the affected area.

WAX JAMBU PRESERVES
Makes about 3 cups

Wax jambu has a rose-infused, green apple flavor that lends itself perfectly to preserves.

INGREDIENTS:

- 4 cups chopped wax jambu fruit

- 1 cup sugar

- 1 pinch ground cinnamon

INSTRUCTIONS:

- Place all ingredients in a heavy saucepan over medium heat, stirring constantly. Cook until syrupy.

USE:

This recipe is delicious served on toast, warmed over ice cream or pancakes, or added to a smoothie

DID YOU KNOW?

In addition to the properties listed, the flowers are astringent. They are made into a syrup used to reduce fevers.

Yarrow

An erect perennial herb, yarrow produces one or more stems of up to 3 feet high. The leaves, which are from 2 to 8 inches in length, are feather-like and arranged spirally on the stems. The ray (three to eight in number) and disc (15 to 40 in number) flowers are white to pink. In antiquity, yarrow was the go-to herb for staunching blood.

WHERE IT CAN BE FOUND:

All 50 US States, all of Canada, throughout Europe, throughout Asia, New Zealand, Central America, Mexico, South America

PROPERTIES AND USE:

Analgesic, anti-aging, antidepressant, anti-inflammatory, antiseptic, antibacterial, expectorant, hepatoprotective, anti-allergen, diuretic, cholagogue, emmenaogue, hypotensive, antispasmodic, antitumor, stomachic, abortifacient. Used to treat sore throat, skin conditions, toothache, candida, incontinence, swelling, thrombosis, catarrh, toothache, migraine, amenorrhea.

TRADITIONAL PREPARATION:

For amenorrhea, catarrh, and allergies, boil 6 tablespoons of the dried leaf in 2 1/2 cups water. **For**

migraine, place leaves in nostrils. This will cause bleeding but relieve pressure. For toothache, chew fresh leaves. **For acne and other skin conditions**, make a decoction of 1/2 cup leaves in 2 cups boiled water; cool and wash with it. You can drink this warm or cool for all conditions. **To stop bleeding on small to moderate-sized cuts**, place a leaf on the affected area. **For larger cuts** (when proper first aid is not available), make a plaster by chewing on several leaves, and gently pushing them into the wound.

Yerba Buena

Yerba Buena is an aromatic perennial herb with woody stems; petioled leaves; and white, lavender, or salmon-colored flowers. It has been used medicinally since ancient times and is a member of the mint family. The Spaniards dubbed it *yerba Buena*, meaning "good herb". It is sometimes called peppermint.

WHERE IT CAN BE FOUND:

Mediterranean, Asia, Australia, Mexico, Central America, South America, Alaska, British Columbia, Washington, Oregon, California, Montana, Idaho

PROPERTIES AND USE:

Expectorant, carminative, stomachic, analgesic, stimulant, antispasmodic, anti-inflammatory, emmenagogue, antiseptic, febrifuge, and treats headache, cough, colds, stomachache, toothache, mouth sores, nausea, dizziness, fainting, insect bites, rheumatism, arthritis, sore muscles, swelling

TRADITIONAL PREPARATION:

For nausea, dizziness, and fainting, bruise fresh leaves and place in the nostrils. For insect bites, rub crushed fresh leaves or juice on the affected area. **For general use**, boil 6 tablespoons chopped fresh leaves in 2 cups water for 15 minutes. Cool, and then strain. Divide into thirds and consume one-third per day. You may also use this as a gargle. **For rheumatism, arthritis, sore muscles, swelling, and headaches**, warm the leaves, and then crush them. Apply to the affected area. The juice from the crushed leaves can also be applied on its own. **For toothaches**, soak a piece of cotton in the sap from a freshly cut stem, and insert it directly into or on the tooth.

DID YOU KNOW?

In 1992, the Department of Health of the Philippines named yerba Buena one of the top 10 medicinal plants.

Yucca

Modern science is just now showing medicinal benefits that have long been known by the medicine men and women of the American Southwest. Yucca contains phytochemicals that work along with the immune system to decrease inflammation in the body. It is a clumped plant with sword-like, sharp leaves, and cream-colored flowers. Other names include Mojave Yucca, Adam's needle, bear grass, soap weed, Spanish bayonet, and Yucca root. Relatives grow throughout the US, as well as in certain areas of Canada.

WHERE IT CAN BE FOUND:

Central America, South America, Caribbean, Arizona, California, Nevada, Utah

PROPERTIES AND USE:

Analgesic, anti-inflammatory, hypotensive, and is used to treat rheumatism, arthritis, sore muscles, headache, intestinal pain, skin conditions, dandruff, hair loss, bleeding, high cholesterol, sores

TRADITIONAL PREPARATION:

Yucca can be purchased in capsule, powder, or extract format. Add the powder to food to mask the strong taste or swallow the capsules so that you don't have to taste it at all. Yucca root can be made into a tea, which is pale yellow in color and best combined with ginseng, licorice, and/or ginger. The root is used to make the powder for natural remedies. It can also be cooked and eaten, and it is often fried.

Sometimes Yucca extract is used as a flavoring and foaming agent in carbonated beverages. Certain compounds have also been used to produce modern medication.

44 Essential Oils and uses

Arborvitae

Is your nose always dripping? Do you have contested sinuses and difficulty breathing? Do you leave a trail of Kleenex wherever you go?

Arborvitae essential oil is the support you need to get through the winter season! Regularly used by the Native Americans, arborvitae oil offers a number of health benefits and additional practical benefits, as well.

For instance, the oil possesses natural preservative properties that help protect against wood rot. In fact, the Arborvitae tree is called the "tree of life," and the wood, itself, lived plenty of life, providing baskets, vessels, totem poles, clothing, and many other goods for the Native Americans.

The oil supplies similar properties when it comes to bodily health by supporting normal cell activity and combatting harmful environmental elements and seasonal threats. This is largely due to its high tropolone content. The oil's strong purifying and cleansing properties, along with its natural ability to repel insects, make it one powerful agent to have on hand when you're venturing out of doors.

Uses:

To cleanse and purify surfaces or hands, add 3-4 drops arborvitae to a spray bottle then fill the rest with distilled water. Shake well and use as needed.

For bodily health, put 1-2 drops on your pulse points to support natural cell function. You can also use arborvitae to scare those bugs away by diffusing the oil throughout the affected area or creating your own bug spray. Lastly, you can apply arborvitae topically to support skin health. Simply rub 1-2 drops softly over the affected area.

General Methods of Application

Apply NEAT. Aromatically. Topically.

Precautions:

Those with sensitive skin should dilute the oil with a carrier oil. Avoid touching the eyes, ears, and other sensitive areas with the oil. People who are nursing, pregnant, or are receiving medical attention should consult their physician before use. Additionally, make sure to store the oil away from children.

Blend Recipe: Wood Preservation Polish
Ingredients:

- 4 drops Arborvitae Essential Oil
- 2 drops Lemon Essential Oil

Directions:

Other surface cleansing uses include applying it to wood for preservation. Blend together the oils and, with a soft rag, polish up that antique rocking chair or bed stand.

Basil

Do you have trouble concentrating? Are you easily distracted?

Try using basil essential oil to help sharpen focus. Often used in cooking, basil offers a number of health benefits whether taken internally or applied aromatically or topically. The oil possesses natural cooling properties when it comes to the skin helping relieve minor skin irritations.

In fact, when applied to the temples and/or the back of the neck, basil can ease tension or stress. The oil supports memory function and enhances alertness, making it perfect for brainwork. Not only does it strengthen the mind and skin, but it also alleviates sore muscles and joints and fortifies healthy and clear breathing.

The oil's strength, along with its versatility, makes it one powerful agent to have on hand when cramming for a test or burning the midnight oil (pun intended).

Uses:

To stimulate memory function and sharpen concentration, add 3-4 drops basil to your diffuser.

You can also use basil to scare those bugs away by diffusing the oil throughout the affected area or creating your own bug spray. Lastly, you can apply basil topically to support skin health or relieve sore muscles and joints. Simply rub 1-2 drops softly over the affected area.

General Methods of Application

Apply NEAT. Aromatically. Internally. Topically.

Precautions:

Those with sensitive skin should dilute the oil with a carrier oil. Avoid touching the eyes, ears, and other sensitive areas with the oil. People who are nursing, pregnant, or are receiving medical attention should consult their physician before use. Additionally, make sure to store the oil away from children.

Blend Recipe: Spider Bite Salve
Ingredients:

- 4 ounces Distilled Water
- 3 drops Basil Essential Oil

- 3 drops Lemon Essential Oil

Directions:

For skin irritation caused by a spider bite, mix all ingredients together into a glass spray bottle. Shake well and spray over the bite. Let air-dry.

Bergamot

Does your skin get angry whenever you eat junk food? Are your breakouts scarring up your complexion so that you can barely recognize yourself? Bergamot oil is the oil for you! Bergamot oil and the citrus plant, itself, are sensitive to soil quality and climate and require strict specifications for cultivation.

Regularly utilized by the Greeks and Italians, bergamot oil offers a number of health benefits that support the mind and body. Bergamot possesses skin-rejuvenating properties that help promote clear skin. The oil has a calming effect to reduce tension and stress, or abating feelings of sadness.

This is largely due to its bright and uplifting scent. The oil's capacity to reduce tension, along with its natural ability to support healthy skin, make it one powerful agent to have on hand when you want to look your best and feel your brightest.

Uses:

To reduce tension, add 3-4 drops bergamot to your diffuser and diffuse regularly. Add a few drops to your bathwater at the end of the day to melt stress away.

For skin health, put 1-2 drops on the area of concern. You can also use a drop or two of bergamot in your tea for a nice citrus flavor. Lastly, you can apply bergamot topically in massage to knead relaxation into your muscles. Simply rub 1-2 drops softly over the affected area.

General Methods of Application

Apply diluted for sensitive skin. Aromatically. Topically. Internally.

Precautions:

Those with sensitive skin should dilute the oil with a carrier oil. Avoid touching the eyes, ears, and other sensitive areas with the oil. People who are nursing, pregnant, or are receiving medical attention should consult their physician before use. Additionally, make sure to store the oil away from children. This oil is photosensitive; avoid direct sunlight for 12 hours after applied topically.

Blend Recipe: Craving Combatant

Ingredients:

- 5 drops Bergamot Essential Oil
- 2 drops Lemon Essential Oil
- 1 drop Ginger Essential Oil
- 1 drop Peppermint Essential Oil
- 2 ounces Jojoba or Almond Oil

Directions:

The next time you're craving that Mars bar, blend together all oils in a small glass bowl. Apply topically to your feet's reflex points. You can also use an aromatic method. Nix the carrier oil and diffuse throughout the room.

Black Pepper

Do all systems malfunction during seasonal changes? For added support, fortify your body with black pepper essential oil! Frequently used to spice up our daily meals, black pepper offers a number of health benefits and supportive properties.

For instance, the oil naturally possesses high levels of antioxidants that help protect against free radicals. The oil supports healthy circulation and combats feelings of anxiety or nerves. This is largely due to its tension relieving properties. The oil's strength makes it a protective aid against seasonal threats, and its support of everything from anxiety to digestion covers many aspects of human health.

Uses:

To soothe muscle and joint tension, dilute 3-4 drops black pepper with a carrier oil and massage into the area of concern. Diffuse or inhale for nerves or feelings of anxiety.

For a digestive aid and seasoning, place 1-2 drops on your soups, salads, or any other dish. You can also use black pepper as a general health enhancer by placing a couple drops in a veggie capsule and taking internally.

General Methods of Application

Apply diluted for sensitive skin. Aromatically. Topically. Internally

Precautions:

Those with sensitive skin should dilute the oil with carrier oil such as fractionated coconut oil. Avoid touching the eyes, ears, and other sensitive areas with the oil. People who are nursing, pregnant, or are receiving medical attention should consult their physician before use. Additionally, make sure to store the oil away from children.

Blend Recipe: Get-Up-&-Go Energy Plus

Ingredients:

- 10 drops Black Pepper Essential Oil
- 10 drops Cinnamon Bark Essential Oil
- 10 drops Wild Orange Essential Oil

Directions:

For a boost of zest and energy, blend these oils together in a small glass bottle. Add 6-7 drops to your diffuser and breathe in. Feel energized and bound for glory!

Cardamom

Do you suffer from occasional digestive problems? Cardamom oil can support mild upset stomach and other digestive problems.

Regularly used to spice up cooked or baked goods, cardamom offers a number of health benefits and supports several areas of overall health. For instance, the oil possesses natural digestion supportive properties that help protect against the occasional feelings of nausea. In fact, the oil can also be used as a seasoning, so the digestive function is built right in.

Cardamom oil supports respiratory health by promoting clear breathing. This is largely due to its high 1,8-cineole content. The oil's strong mood-enhancing properties, along with its natural ability to aid digestion,   make it one powerful agent to have on hand when you need an uplifting aroma to better your mood or a topical application to settle your stomach.

Uses:

To aid gastrointestinal function and season all variety of dishes, add 1-2 drops to your food or drink and take internally.

For respiratory health, put 1-2 drops on your chest and massage toward the throat. You can also use cardamom to relieve the occasional bout of motion sickness or upset stomach by diffusing the oil throughout or inhaling directly.

General Methods of Application

Apply NEAT. Aromatically. Internally. Topically.

Precautions:

Those with sensitive skin should dilute the oil with a carrier oil. Avoid touching the eyes, ears, and other sensitive areas with the oil. People who are nursing, pregnant, or are receiving medical attention should consult their physician before use. Additionally, make sure to store the oil away from children.

Blend Recipe: Mild Constipation Relief

Ingredients:

- 15 drops Patchouli Essential Oil
- 5 drops Cardamom Essential Oil

- 5 drops Black Pepper Essential Oil
- 2 Tbsp Sweet Almond Oil

Directions:

To support gastrointestinal issues, like mild, occasional constipation, combine ingredients in a small glass bottle and mix until well blended. Apply a few drops of this blend to the lower abdomen, massaging in a clockwise motion.

Cassia

Do your hands and feet get cold quickly? Is circulation a major concern in your book?

Use cassia to pump up your blood flow. Frequently used as a substitute for cinnamon, cassia oil offers as many health benefits and supportive properties as its sister.

For instance, the oil possesses natural immune stimulant properties that help protect against environmental threats. The oil supports digestive health and promotes circulation, which enables it to relieve sore and achy joints.

The oil's powerful properties, along with its natural ability to uplift per its warm aroma, make it one powerful agent to have on hand during seasonal changes or whenever your immune function may need a boost.

Uses:

To enhance immune function, add 1-2 drops cassia to a veggie capsule and take once a day.

For digestive health, blend 1-2 drops cassia with 1-2 drops lemon in your drinking water and take internally. This can also be used to calm cravings and relieve hunger. Lastly, you can apply cassia topically to support achy muscles and joints. Simply dilute 1-2 drops and rub softly over the affected area.

General Methods of Application

Apply diluted. Aromatically. Topically. Internally.

Precautions:

Those with sensitive skin should dilute the oil with a carrier oil. Avoid touching the eyes, ears, and other sensitive areas with the oil. People who are nursing, pregnant, or are receiving medical attention should consult their physician before use. Additionally, make sure to store the oil away from children.

Blend Recipe: Festive Cheer Room Spray

Ingredients:

- 1 Tbsp Pure Vanilla Extract
- 3 drops Cassia Essential Oil
- 3 drops Clove Essential Oil
- 3 drops Wild Orange Essential Oil
- Distilled or Tap Water

Directions:

Uplift your spirits with a warm and cheery room spray during the holiday season by simply combining all ingredients in an 8 once glass spray bottle, filling the remainder with distilled water. Shake vigorously to blend and spray in the air as needed.

Cedarwood

Is breathing a struggle? Is a short walk between rooms or to the mailbox leave you panting for air?

Cedarwood essential oil is your guardian angel. Often used as a promoter of wellness and vitality, cedarwood oil offers a number of versatile health benefits.

For instance, the oil possesses natural warming properties that helped support the large cedarwood trees from whence it came, which are native to cold high altitudes. This warming ability transfers to the human body, in a sense, aiding respiratory function.

The oil supports healthy and clear skin, while its scent relaxes. Cedarwood's soothing properties, along with its natural ability to repel insects, make it one powerful agent to have on hand when you're venturing out of doors.

Uses:

To fortify respiratory function, add 3-4 drops to your diffuser or breathe in directly. You can also add a few drops to your diffuser simply for relaxation.

For skin health, add 1-2 drops to your daily facial moisturizer and use as normal. Lastly, you can apply cedarwood topically in massage. Simply dilute 1-2 drops with a carrier oil and rub softly over the affected area.

General Methods of Application

Apply diluted for sensitive skin. Aromatically. Topically.

Precautions:

Those with sensitive skin should dilute the oil with a carrier oil. Avoid touching the eyes, ears, and other sensitive areas with the oil. People who are nursing, pregnant, or are receiving medical attention should consult their physician before use. Additionally, make sure to store the oil away from children.

Blend Recipe: Woodsy Insect Repellent
Ingredients:

- 3.5 ounces Distilled Water
- 13 drops Cedarwood Essential Oil
- 10 drops Lavender Essential Oil
- 6 drops Eucalyptus Essential Oil
- 5 drops Lemongrass Essential Oil
- 4 drops Peppermint Essential Oil

Directions:

For an effective woodsy scented insect repellent, combine all ingredients in a glass spray bottle. Shake vigorously to mix. Spray over exposed skin whenever you're headed outside. Shake well before each use.

Cilantro

Tummy growling even when you aren't hungry?

Are bowel movements irregular? Cilantro can help you stay regular. Often utilized for culinary purposes, cilantro offers a versatile range of health benefits.

For instance, the oil possesses natural cleansing and detoxifying properties partially due to its high antioxidant content. In fact, when added to salads, meat entrees, and dips, like guacamole, not only does your cooking benefit from the fresh cilantro flavor, but also you're absorbing these protective antioxidants, which rid of free radicals.

Cilantro oil supports digestive function, helping to relieve the occasional upset stomach. Cilantro's strong purifying and cleansing properties, along with its natural capacity to support the skin,   make it one powerful agent to have on hand when shopping for multi-purpose oils.

Uses:

To cleanse and detoxify the body, add 1-2 drops cilantro to your drinking water and take internally.

For digestive health, put 1-2 drops in your meals. You can also use cilantro in a diffusion blend with citrus oils. Lastly, you can apply cilantro topically to support skin health. Simply rub 1-2 drops softly over the affected area.

General Methods of Application

Apply NEAT. Aromatically. Topically. Internally

Precautions:

Those with sensitive skin should dilute the oil with a carrier oil. Avoid touching the eyes, ears, and other sensitive areas with the oil. People who are nursing, pregnant, or are receiving medical attention should consult their physician before use. Additionally, make sure to store the oil away from children.

Blend Recipe: Relief from Occasional Upset Stomach
Ingredients:

- 1 drop Cilantro Essential Oil
- 1 drop Rosemary Essential Oil
- ½ glass Warm Drinking Water

Directions:

To relieve occasional upset stomach and support digestive function, combine the oils in a warm glass of drinking water. Mix well and drink.

Cinnamon Bark

Do you prefer to use natural solutions for cleaning products? Maybe not, yet, but it's a consideration.

Most consumer cleaning products are full of highly toxic chemicals. There are simpler, and safer cleaning solutions. Consider cinnamon bark essential oil for your cleansing needs.

Frequently used for culinary purposes, especially in baking or hot drinks, cinnamon bark offers a number of health benefits and is one of the more versatile oils. For instance, the oil possesses high levels of cinnamaldehyde that help protect the immune system.

In fact, cinnamon bark has long been used for its internal benefits, like its ability to stimulate healthy circulation. The oil helps to relieve occasional sore muscles and joints, while also serving as a strong cleanser that combats bacterial threats.

The oil's strong purifying and cleansing properties also extend to oral health and, along with its natural ability to boost the immune system, these components make cinnamon bark one powerful agent to have on hand at nearly any turn.

Uses:

To cleanse and purify surfaces, add 3-4 drops cinnamon to a spray bottle then fill the rest with distilled water. Shake well and use as needed.

Add a drop to your toothbrush before the paste to supplement oral health. For immune system health, put 2 drops of cinnamon in a veggie capsule and take internally. You can also use cinnamon bark to soothe your throat by adding a drop to hot tea. Lastly, you can dilute cinnamon and apply it topically to support sore muscles and joints. Simply rub softly over the affected area.

General Methods of Application

Apply diluted. Aromatically. Topically. Internally

Precautions:

Always dilute the oil with a carrier oil. Avoid touching the eyes, ears, and other sensitive areas with the oil. People who are nursing, pregnant, or are receiving medical attention should consult their physician before use. Additionally, make sure to store the oil away from children.

Blend Recipe: Immune Supportive Massage Blend

Ingredients:

- 5 drops Melissa Essential Oil
- 10 drops Rosemary Essential Oil

- 10 drops Eucalyptus Essential Oil
- 15 drops Cinnamon Essential Oil
- 15 drops Oregano Essential Oil
- 15 drops Black Pepper Essential Oil
- 20 drops Clove Bud Essential Oil
- 30 drops Wild Orange Essential Oil
- 6 mL Coconut Oil

Directions:

For an immune boosting massage blend, combine all ingredients in a small glass jar. Blend well and apply topically, as needed. Massage into the body's reflex points whenever your immune system is weak.

Clary Sage

Do you struggle with hormonal fluctuation during your monthly period or with menopause?

Hormones can wreak havoc on your emotions and bodily functions. Fortunately, there's clary sage.

Regularly used for women's health issues, clary sage offers a number of health benefits, especially those involving hormone balance. For instance, the oil possesses natural properties that help regulate issues associated with menstruation. This is because the oil has a high content of linalyl acetate, which is a member of the ester group.

The oil supplies helps relieve nervous tension and is a fantastic skin support and soothing agent. Clary sage's ability to support feminine discomfort, along with its natural hormone-balancing properties, make it one powerful agent to have on hand when you need to lighten the mood and support fluctuation.

Uses:

To calm menstrual discomfort, put 3-4 drops clary sage on the lower abdomen. Massage gently into the stomach. Mix a couple drops each of clary sage and Roman chamomile in your bathwater for a calming and stress-relieving bath.

For hair and scalp health, put 1-2 drops into your daily dose of shampoo. You can also use clary sage aromatically to relax and improve sleep. Lastly, you can apply clary sage topically to support skin health. Simply rub 1-2 drops softly over the affected area.

General Methods of Application

Apply NEAT. Aromatically. Topically.

Precautions:

Those with sensitive skin should dilute the oil with a carrier oil. Avoid touching the eyes, ears, and other sensitive areas with the oil. People who are nursing, pregnant, or are receiving medical attention should consult their physician before use. Additionally, make sure to store the oil away from children.

Blend Recipe: Hot Flash Relief

Ingredients:

- 3 ounces Distilled Water
- 1 drop Peppermint Essential Oil
- 2 drops Patchouli Essential Oil

- 2 drops Clary Sage Essential Oil

Directions:

Use this blend when you're going through menopause to help relieve the occasional hot flash. Simply blend all ingredients in a 4-ounce glass spray bottle. Shake it up and spritz over your chest, face or other areas of concern whenever needed.

Clove Bud

Frequently used in traditional oral health, clove bud offers a number of versatile health benefits.

For instance, the oil possesses natural hygiene supporting properties that help protect the gums and teeth. The oil supports heart health by boosting blood circulation. This is largely due to its high eugenol content.

Moreover, clove bud is high in antioxidants, which combat free radicals in the body, allowing it to support the immune system and overall bodily functions. The oil's strong energizing properties, along with its natural ability to protect, make it one powerful agent to have on hand when your immune system has taken a hit.

Uses:

Add a drop to your toothbrush before the paste to supplement oral health. Relieve toothaches or gum sensitivity with a drop of clove applied to the area of concern.

For immune system health, put 2 drops of clove bud in a veggie capsule and take internally. You can also use clove bud to soothe your throat by adding a drop to the back of the tongue.

General Methods of Application

Apply diluted. Aromatically. Topically. Internally.

Precautions:

Always dilute the oil with a carrier oil. Avoid touching the eyes, ears, and other sensitive areas with the oil. People who are nursing, pregnant, or are receiving medical attention should consult their physician before use. Additionally, make sure to store the oil away from children.

Blend Recipe: Germs-Be-Gone Diffusion Blend
Ingredients:

- 3 drops Clove Bud Essential Oil
- 3 drops Tea Tree Essential Oil
- 3 drops Lemongrass Essential Oil

Directions:

Tackle germs throughout your home or office by blending all ingredients in your diffuser. Use as normal to clear the air and breathe in deeply for aromatic support.

Coriander

Coriander supports a healthy digestive tract simply by adding to your meals.

Coriander oil is a multi-purpose oil that offers a number of health benefits. For instance, the oil possesses natural digestive properties that help protect against stomach upset and even assist in maintaining healthy insulin levels.

The oil benefits skin health by reducing oil production and, thereby, breakouts. Moreover, coriander can help ease discomfort in achy muscles and joints, while relieving tension in massage therapy. Coriander oil's capable properties, along with its natural ability to aid digestion, make it one powerful agent to have on hand during mealtime or, really, any time your skin, muscles, and joints need a leg-up.

Uses:

To relieve occasional digestive issues, apply topically to the abdomen in gentle massage or add 1-2 drops coriander to your drinking water. Combine a coriander protocol with the use of Slim & Sassy for assistance in maintaining healthy insulin levels.

For skin health, put 1-2 drops overtop any area of concern. Lastly, you can apply coriander topically to support muscles and joints. Simply rub 1-2 drops gently over the affected area.

General Methods of Application

Apply NEAT. Aromatically. Internally. Topically.

Precautions:

Those with sensitive skin should dilute the oil with a carrier oil. Avoid touching the eyes, ears, and other sensitive areas with the oil. People who are nursing, pregnant, or are receiving medical attention should consult their physician before use. Additionally, make sure to store the oil away from children.

Blend Recipe: Energy Stimulating Massage
Ingredients:

- 175 mL Almond Carrier Oil
- 10 drops Lime Essential Oil

- 12 drops Sandalwood Essential Oil
- 12 drops Bergamot Essential Oil
- 15 drops Coriander Essential Oil

Directions:

For massage that uplifts and boosts energy, blend all oils in a small glass jar until well combined. Apply as normal in a full-body massage or into the body's reflex points. Store the remainder in a cool, dry place for future use.

Cypress

Breathing is a problem for many people. Any number of illnesses or disorders make taking in oxygen a chore.

Cypress oil will open up your airways, enabling a much more restful sleep. Regularly utilized in massage therapy, cypress oil provides a fresh, clean scent, alongside a number of health benefits.

For instance, the oil offers natural tension-relieving properties that help soothe muscles and joints. Cypress supports a healthy respiratory tract and clear breathing, while promoting skin health.

Additionally, the oil promotes localized blood flow, which supports the body's circulation. Cypress oil's effective properties, along with its natural ability to soothe and calm, make it one powerful agent to have on hand when you're in need of balancing and mental grounding.

Uses:

To support proper breathing and respiratory health, add 3-4 drops cypress to a carrier oil then apply over the chest. For muscle and joint discomfort, apply topically, massaging over the area of concern.

For throat discomfort, inhale, diffuse, or gargle with cypress (make sure to spit out!). You can also use cypress to firm up and tone the skin by combining it with grapefruit essential oil and a carrier oil and applying topically. Lastly, you can apply cypress topically on its own to support general skin health. Simply rub 1-2 drops softly over the affected area.

General Methods of Application

Apply NEAT. Aromatically. Topically.

Precautions:

Those with sensitive skin should dilute the oil with a carrier oil. Avoid touching the eyes, ears, and other sensitive areas with the oil. People who are nursing, pregnant, or are receiving medical attention should consult their physician before use. Additionally, make sure to store the oil away from children.

Blend Recipe: Circulation Support
Ingredients:

- ½ ounce Coconut Oil
- 4 drops Cypress Essential Oil
- 2 drops Wild Orange Essential Oil
- 2 drops Rosemary Essential Oil
- 2 drops Cilantro Essential Oil

Directions:

To help regulate healthy blood circulation, blend all ingredients in a small glass jar until well combined. Apply a small amount to the reflex points and the ankles, stroking towards the heart. Store the remainder in a cool, dry place.

Eucalyptus

Eucalyptus essential oil may well be the first essential oil you ever experienced. It is often used to clear clear breathing and fortify respiratory function; eucalyptus oil offers a number of health benefits.

For instance, the oil possesses natural cleansing and purifying properties that help protect against environmental threats.

Eucalyptus oil supports immune system function, which is essential when there are seasonal hazards. The oil can be used to fortify oral health (dilute with water and use as a gargle, not to be taken internally).

Moreover, eucalyptus can help soothe and relieve muscle soreness and fatigue, while reducing stress. The oil's strong purifying and cleansing properties, along with its natural ability to serve respiratory health, make it one powerful agent to have on hand when there are harmful environmental threats.

Uses:

To cleanse and purify surfaces, add 3-4 drops eucalyptus to a spray bottle then fill the rest with distilled water. Shake well and use as needed. Add lemon and peppermint for a super blend.

For respiratory health, blend 1-2 drops with a carrier oil and massage over the chest. You can also use the cup and inhale protocol, which involves adding 1-2 drops to your hands, rubbing them together, cupping your nose, and inhaling slowly and deeply. Additionally, for clear breathing pathways, add a few drops to a steam shower.

General Methods of Application

Apply diluted for sensitive skin. Aromatically. Topically.

Precautions:

Those with sensitive skin should dilute the oil with a carrier oil. Avoid touching the eyes, ears, and other sensitive areas with the oil. People who are nursing, pregnant, or are receiving medical attention should consult their physician before use. Additionally, make sure to store the oil away from children.

Blend Recipe: Easy Breathing Diffusion Blend

Ingredients:

- 1 drop Eucalyptus Essential Oil
- 1 drop Rosemary Essential oil
- 1 drop Lime Essential Oil
- 1 drop Peppermint Essential Oil
- 1 drop Lemon Essential Oil

Directions:

Fortify the respiratory system with this clear breathing diffusion blend. Simply combine all oils in your diffuser and inhale deeply.

Fennel

Add fennel to your meals for Relieves occasional indigestion and digestive troubles. Often used by Roman warriors, fennel was believed to fortify the mind and body for war. The oil possesses natural digestive properties that help protect against issues like occasional indigestion.

Fennel is effective in relieving all sorts of stomachaches, even those caused by menstrual cramps. The oil calms minor skin irritations and strengthens the lymphatic system. Fennel's strong digestive properties, along with its natural ability to support the skin, make it one powerful agent to have on hand when you're in need of relief.

Uses:

To support digestion or menstrual issues, blend 3-4 drops with a carrier oil and massage over the affected area and into the soles of the feet. You can also take internally if you're experiencing a minor stomachache by placing a couple drops in your hot tea.

To use as a flavoring agent, put 1-2 drops in your dish (particularly good in desserts). You can also use fennel to calm cravings by placing a drop below the tongue.

General Methods of Application

Apply diluted for sensitive skin. Aromatically. Topically. Internally.

Precautions:

Those with sensitive skin should dilute the oil with a carrier oil. Avoid touching the eyes, ears, and other sensitive areas with

the oil. People who are nursing, pregnant, or are receiving medical attention should consult their physician before use. Additionally, make sure to store the oil away from children.

Blend Recipe: Relief for Occasional Constipation
Ingredients:

- 1 drop Ginger Essential Oil
- 2 drops Fennel Essential Oil
- 2 drops Peppermint Essential Oil

Directions:

If you experience occasional constipation, you can relieve it through an essential oil capsule. Simply add all ingredients in a "00" veggie capsule and, every three hours, ingest until the issue is resolved.

Frankincense

Is your skin tone and condition disappointing/ Essential oils can help, and particularly frankincense. Regularly used by the ancient Egyptians, frankincense oil offers a number of health benefits when it comes to skin health.

For instance, the oil possesses natural rejuvenating properties that help protect against blemishes and aging skin. In fact, the oil is a supporter of cellular function, which protects the appearance of the skin and fortifies overall bodily function. The oil reinvigorates the immune system, helping to maintain it to defend against environmental threats. The oil's incomparable properties, along with its natural ability to fortify the skin, make it one powerful agent to have on hand in nearly any scenario.

Uses:

To support younger-looking skin, add 3-4 drops frankincense to the area of concern. You can also strengthen nails by applying a drop topically to the nail's surface.

For bodily health, put 1-2 drops on your pulse points to support natural cell function. You can also use frankincense for relaxation and mood support by massaging the oil into the soles of the feet.

General Methods of Application

Apply NEAT. Aromatically. Internally. Topically.

Precautions:

Those with sensitive skin should dilute the oil with a carrier oil. Avoid touching the eyes, ears, and other sensitive areas with the oil. People who are nursing, pregnant, or are receiving medical attention should consult their physician before use. Additionally, make sure to store the oil away from children.

Blend Recipe: Strong Nails

Ingredients:

- 2 drops Frankincense Essential Oil
- 2 drops Lemon Essential Oil
- 2 drops Myrrh Essential Oil
- 1 drop Wintergreen Essential Oil
- 4 drops Wheat Germ

Directions:

Blend all ingredients in a small glass jar until well combined. Apply 1 drop of the blend to each nail, massaging into the cuticle and nail. Do this 2-3 times daily.

Geranium

Are you ashamed of blemishes on your skin? Do you want to defy visible aging? Geranium essential oil is for you. Frequently used by the ancient Egyptians, geranium oil offers a number of health benefits to fortify skin.

Geranium oil offers natural rejuvenating properties that help protect against skin irritations and aging. In fact, geranium oil supports clear, healthy, younger-looking skin that's radiant and firm. The oil supports liver function, while relieving stress and occasional nervousness. The oil's strong and age-defying properties, along with its natural ability to promote joy, make it one powerful agent to have on hand when you want to look as young as you feel.

Uses:

To promote radiant-looking skin, add 3-4 drops geranium to a pan of hot steaming water, place a towel over your head, and have yourself a steam facial. You can also place a drop into your daily moisturizer and use to combat oily skin

For hair health, put 2-3 drops in your shampoo each use. You can also diffuse for stress relief.

General Methods of Application

Apply diluted for sensitive skin. Aromatically. Topically. Internally.

Precautions:

Those with sensitive skin should dilute the oil with a carrier oil. Avoid touching the eyes, ears, and other sensitive areas with the oil. People who are nursing, pregnant, or are receiving medical attention should consult their physician before use. Additionally, make sure to store the oil away from children.

Blend Recipe: Age-defying Salve

Ingredients:

- 1 ounce Carrier Oil
- 4 drops Geranium Essential Oil
- 3 drops Lavender Essential Oil
- 3 drops Patchouli Essential Oil
- 2 drops Frankincense Essential Oil

Directions:

Promote smoother, firmer skin and diminish signs of wrinkles by blending all oils in a small glass jar. Twice a day – morning and night – dab over areas of concern, along with your daily skincare regimen.

Ginger

Ginger can help your digestive system establish regularity. Often used in cooking, especially in Asia, ginger offers health benefits primarily that serve digestion. For instance, the oil possesses natural soothing and relieving properties that help calm occasional nausea, upset stomach, or motion sickness.

In fact, carrying the bottle on a long road trip or a rocking boat can ease the most sensitive stomach.

The oil's strong digestive properties, along with its natural ability to flavor everything from baked goods to stir fry dishes, make it one powerful agent to have on hand when you're throwing together a meal.

Uses:

To relieve the occasional upset stomach, add 1-2 drops ginger to a glass of drinking water and take internally. For motion sickness or nausea, add a drop or two to your hands, cup and inhale, for stomach-calming relief.

To serve the digestive tract, dilute 1-2 drops with a carrier oil and apply topically to the stomach and the soles of the feet. Lastly, you can add ginger oil to any number of dishes for its pungent and spicy flavor.

General Methods of Application

Apply diluted for sensitive skin. Aromatically. Topically. Internally.

Precautions:

Those with sensitive skin should dilute the oil with a carrier oil. Avoid touching the eyes, ears, and other sensitive areas with the oil. People who are nursing, pregnant, or are receiving medical attention should consult their physician before use. Additionally, make sure to store the oil away from children.

Blend Recipe: Morning Sickness Relief
Ingredients:

- 8 ounces Drinking Water
- 1 drop Ginger Essential Oil
- 1 drop Lemon Essential Oil
- 1 tsp Honey

Directions:

Relieve morning sickness with this tasty and stomach-calming blend. Simply stir all ingredients in a glass and drink each morning, right when you get up.

Grapefruit

Are you feeling the blues? Do you wish you had more energy and a positive outlook on life? Grapefruit will be a burst of sunlight on a cloudy day!

Often referred to as the "forbidden fruit", grapefruit offers a number of health benefits that fortify overall health. For instance, the oil possesses natural purifying and cleansing properties that help protect against skin problems.

Grapefruit oil is also said to support proper metabolic function, which can strengthen your ability to stay healthy and fit. The oil soothes sore muscles and joints, while combatting physical and mental fatigue. The oil's strong purifying and cleansing properties, along with its natural ability to invigorate, make it one powerful agent to have on hand when you're gearing up to get in shape.

Uses:

To sharpen focus, add 3-4 drops grapefruit to a diffuser and inhale deeply. You can also use grapefruit topically for minor skin issues and bug bites. Simply dilute and apply it to the area of concern.

For muscle and joint discomfort, massage 1-2 drops gently into the affected area. You can also use grapefruit to clear up breathing through diffusion or a topical application to the chest.

General Methods of Application

Apply NEAT. Aromatically. Internally. Topically.

Precautions:

Those with sensitive skin should dilute the oil with a carrier oil. Avoid touching the eyes, ears, and other sensitive areas with the oil. People who are nursing, pregnant, or are receiving medical attention should consult their physician before use. Additionally, make sure to store the oil away from children. This oil is photosensitive; avoid direct sunlight for 12 hours after applied topically.

Blend Recipe: Detox Massage Blend

Ingredients:

- 30 mL Carrier Oil
- 2 drops Grapefruit Essential Oil
- 2 drops Cypress Essential Oil

- 2 drops Juniper Berry Essential Oil
- 2 drops Lavender Essential Oil
- 2 drops Basil Essential Oil

Directions:

Boost circulation and flush out bodily toxins by combining all oils in a small dark glass jar. Mix or shake well then apply to the reflex points of the feet and over the area of the liver. Store in a cool, dry place and shake well before each use.

Hawaiian Sandalwood

Do those blemishes and spotty complexion leave you feeling embarrassed? Sandalwood oil has come to save the day! Regularly utilized for skin support, sandalwood oil offers a number of health benefits to aid many issues.

For instance, the oil possesses natural properties that help protect against skin aging, including reducing the appearance of scars and blemishes. In fact, sandalwood is a strong supporter of smooth and healthy skin. The oil is supportive of mood and emotion, calming tension and stress, while uplifting and grounding. The oil's strong skin-supportive properties, along with its natural ability to calm the mind, make it one powerful agent to have on hand when you're meditating or looking after the health of your skin.

Uses:

To promote glowing and younger-looking skin, add 1-2 drops sandalwood to your daily skincare regiment and apply as normal.

For stress relief, put 1-2 drops of sandalwood in your bath water and soak the stress away. Breathe in the aroma while you soak. You can also use sandalwood to ease sleep. Either diffuse throughout your bedroom or massage into your back, shoulders, and neck before bedtime.

General Methods of Application

Apply NEAT. Aromatically. Internally. Topically.

Precautions:

Those with sensitive skin should dilute the oil with a carrier oil. Avoid touching the eyes, ears, and other sensitive areas with the oil. People who are nursing, pregnant, or are receiving medical attention should consult their physician before use. Additionally, make sure to store the oil away from children.

Blend Recipe: Scar-reducing Salve
Ingredients:

- 1 Tbsp Grapeseed Oil
- 2 drops Sandalwood Essential Oil
- 4 drops Lavender Essential Oil
- 6 drops Myrrh Essential Oil
- 6 drops Helichrysum Essential Oil

Directions:

Fade away scars or blemishes with this scar-reducing salve. In a small glass jar or container, mix in all oils until well blended. Dab a little over the area of concern, and let the oils soak into your skin. Store the remainder in a cool, dry place and use as needed.

Helichrysum

Are the signs of age showing on your skin? Essential oils can help, and particularly helichrysum. Frequently used by the ancient Greeks, helichrysum offers a number of health benefits and was once called the "Immortal Flower."

For instance, the oil possesses natural skin supportive properties that help reduce the signs of blemishes, scarring, and skin aging. In fact, the oil is a detoxifying agent, helping to strengthen liver function, which affects everything from skin health to brain health. Helichrysum enhances blood flow and is especially supportive of localized circulation. The oil's strong detoxifying properties, along with its natural ability to support the skin and relieve tension, make it one powerful agent to have on hand in any number of scenarios.

Uses:

To cleanse and purify the body, add 1-2 drops helichrysum to every glass of drinking water and ingest regularly.

For skin health, put 1-2 drops over the area of concern, whether wrinkles, blemishes, or scars. You can also use helichrysum to calm stress and tension by diluting the oil for a massage. Apply to the back of the neck, the shoulders, the temples, and the soles of the feet.

General Methods of Application

Apply NEAT. Aromatically. Internally. Topically.

Precautions:

Those with sensitive skin should dilute the oil with a carrier oil. Avoid touching the eyes, ears, and other sensitive areas with the oil. People who are nursing, pregnant, or are receiving medical attention should consult their physician before use. Additionally, make sure to store the oil away from children.

Blend Recipe: Vanquish Varicose Veins

Ingredients:

- 3-4 drops Basil Essential Oil
- 1 drop Helichrysum Essential Oil
- 1 drop Cypress Essential Oil
- 1 drop Wintergreen Essential Oil
- 2 Tsp Carrier Oil

Directions:

To diminish the appearance of varicose veins, blend all ingredients in a small glass jar until well combined, and apply topically to the area of concern, stroking toward the heart. Store the remainder in a cool, dry place.

Jasmine

Do menstrual or hormonal changes disrupt your life? Hormones can wreak havoc on your emotions and add to the drama of the day. Fortunately, there's jasmine. Frequently requiring a labor-intensive cultivation, jasmine oil offers a number of health benefits. For instance, the oil possesses natural nourishing properties that help serve and protect the skin and scalp.

The oil supports emotional wellness by improving confidence and promoting joy. Additionally, jasmine fortifies hormone balance, which helps manage symptoms of PMS. The oil's strong nourishing properties, along with its natural ability to support women's issues, make it one powerful agent to have on hand when your skin is cracking.

Uses:

To regulate symptoms of PMS, apply 3-4 drops jasmine topically to the abdomen and massage in. You can also support hair health by adding a couple drops to your regular conditioning regimen.

For nervous tension, put 1-2 drops on your pulse points to support natural cell function. Lastly, you can apply jasmine topically to support skin health. Simply rub 1-2 drops softly over the affected area.

General Methods of Application

Apply NEAT. Aromatically. Topically.

Precautions:

Those with sensitive skin should dilute the oil with a carrier oil. Avoid touching the eyes, ears, and other sensitive areas with the oil. People who are nursing, pregnant, or are receiving medical attention should consult their physician before use. Additionally, make sure to store the oil away from children.

Blend Recipe: Scent of the Orient Body Wash

Ingredients:

- 2/3 cup Liquid Castile Soap
- ¼ cup Honey
- 2 tsps Sweet Almond Oil
- 1 tsp Vitamin E
- 10 drops Lime Essential Oil
- 20 drops Jasmine Essential Oil

- 25 drops Patchouli Essential Oil

Directions:

For a sweet-smelling bath wash, melt the coconut oil over low heat until smooth. Remove the oil from heat and blend in the honey, vitamin E, and essential oils. Whisk until well combined. Slowly add in the castile soap (warning: will suds up, so stir slowly). Once well blended, pour the liquid soap into a glass bottle and shake well. Use as normal. Always shake before use.

Juniper Berry

Are you ready to flush out your body of all the unnecessary elements and start anew? Juniper berry acts as a natural cleansing and detoxifying agent. Often used for its detoxifying and cleansing properties, juniper berry oil offers a number of health benefits.

For instance, the oil helps rid the body of free radicals by supporting kidney and urinary health. In fact, this capacity to flush out toxins also enables juniper berry to strengthen the skin. The oil calms stress and tension, aromatically, topically, or internally. Juniper berry's strong stress-relieving properties, along with its natural ability to nurture the skin, make it one powerful agent to have on hand when you're in need of a skin or emotional strengthener.

Uses:

To relieve stress and tension, add 3-4 drops juniper berry to your running bathwater to disperse. Melt in your stress-relieving bath, breathing in the soothing aroma.

For detoxification, put 1-2 drops of juniper berry in your drinking water and ingest. Lastly, you can apply juniper berry topically to support skin health. Simply rub 1-2 drops softly over the affected area.

General Methods of Application

Apply NEAT. Aromatically. Internally. Topically.

Precautions:

Those with sensitive skin should dilute the oil with a carrier oil. Avoid touching the eyes, ears, and other sensitive areas with

the oil. People who are nursing, pregnant, or are receiving medical attention should consult their physician before use. Additionally, make sure to store the oil away from children.

Blend Recipe: Skin-Fortifying Hand Sanitizer
Ingredients:

- 1 Tbsp Coconut Oil
- 1.5 ounces Aloe Vera Gel
- 6 drops Clove Essential Oil
- 10 drops Juniper Berry Essential Oil
- 16 drops Lavender Essential Oil

Directions:

To fortify the skin and combat contagions, blend ingredients in a 2 ounce glass bottle until well combined. Apply to your hands on-the-go (no need for water), shaking the bottle before each use.

Lavender

Are you in need of calm, quiet, and peace of mind? Do you struggle with stress and feelings of angst? Lavender is widely used for its calming and relaxing qualities. Regularly used by the ancient Romans and Egyptians, lavender oil offers a number of health benefits when it comes to calming.

For instance, the oil possesses natural stress-relieving properties that help protect against anxious feelings and promote relaxing energies. In fact, lavender brings these soothing elements to skin health, relieving skin irritations and minor skin issues. The oil supplies similar properties when it comes to muscle discomfort, easing strain and tension. Lavender's strong calming properties, along with its natural ability to relieve skin problems and muscle stress, make it one powerful agent to have on hand when you're in need of relaxation.

Uses:

To ease sleep, add 1-2 drops lavender to your pillows and linens or massage into the soles of the feet. You can also add a drop or two to teas, desserts, baked goods, or marinades for a soothing flavor.

For muscle support, rub 1-2 drops into the area of concern. You can also use lavender in a homemade spray to scent closets or your car with the pleasant aroma. Lastly, you can apply lavender topically to support skin health. Simply rub 1-2 drops softly over the affected area.

General Methods of Application

Apply NEAT. Aromatically. Internally. Topically

Precautions:

Those with sensitive skin should dilute the oil with a carrier oil. Avoid touching the eyes, ears, and other sensitive areas with the oil. People who are nursing, pregnant, or are receiving medical attention should consult their physician before use. Additionally, make sure to store the oil away from children.

Blend Recipe: Pillow Spray

Ingredients:

- 15 mL Distilled Water
- 2 drops Lavender Essential Oil

- 1 drop Roman Chamomile Essential Oil
- 1 drop Wild Orange Essential Oil
- 1 drop Ylang Ylang Essential Oil

Directions:

Promote relaxation, calm, and dreamless sleep by blending all ingredients in a glass spray bottle. Shake well to combine and spritz over your linen and pillowcases every night before bedtime.

Lemon

People are looking for alternatives to cleaning products that are environmentally unsound and full of man-made chemicals. Perhaps that sounds like you. Consumer cleaning products are full of highly toxic spliced-together chemicals.

Consider lemon essential oil for your cleansing needs. Frequently used for its cleansing and disinfecting properties, lemon oil offers a number of health benefits that cover a versatile range of issues. For instance, the oil possesses natural purifying properties.

Lemon oil promotes a positive mood and cognitive ability. This is all largely due to its high d-limonene content. Moreover, lemon promotes digestive and respiratory health, serving to relieve minor throat irritations. The oil's strong purifying and cleansing properties, along with its natural ability to promote positivity, make it one powerful agent to have on hand when facing any number of threats in your environment.

Uses:

To cleanse and purify surfaces or hands, add 3-4 drops lemon to a spray bottle then fill the rest with distilled water. Shake well and use as needed. You can also simply apply a few drops lemon to a wet cloth and use it to clean and preserve leather furniture or remove tarnish from silver. When combined with olive oil, the blend is a superb wood polish.

For bodily health, diffuse lemon essential oil to promote respiratory function or mental health.

General Methods of Application

Apply NEAT. Aromatically. Internally. Topically

Precautions:

Those with sensitive skin should dilute the oil with a carrier oil. Avoid touching the eyes, ears, and other sensitive areas with the oil. People who are nursing, pregnant, or are receiving medical attention should consult their physician before use. Additionally, make sure to store the oil away from children. This oil is photosensitive; avoid direct sunlight for 12 hours after applied topically.

Blend Recipe: Disinfecting Spray

Ingredients:

- 1 drop Clary Sage Essential Oil
- 3 drops Lemon Essential Oil
- 3 drops Lime Essential Oil
- 3 drops Wild Orange Essential Oil
- 3 drops Lavender Essential Oil
- 2 ounces Witch Hazel

Directions:

This spray can be used to disinfect and clean surfaces of dust and environmental threats. In a 2 ounce glass spray bottle blend all the ingredients and shake well. Spritz over surfaces and wipe with a rag, as normal. Shake well before each use.

Lemongrass

Often used in Asia to flavor culinary dishes and teas, lemongrass offers a number of health benefits. For instance, the oil possesses natural digestive properties that help protect against the odd stomach upset. Lemongrass also serves to relieve aching muscles and joints, which make it an effective aid for strain and tension.

The oil supports skin, particularly when it comes to purifying and toning. Additionally, lemongrass increases awareness and promotes a positive outlook. The oil's strong digestive properties, along with its natural ability to repel insects, make it one powerful agent to have on hand when you're venturing out of doors.

Uses:

To support digestive health, add 1-2 drops lemongrass to your food or drink. You can also clean and strengthen nails by blending it with melaleuca and applying a drop to each nail.

For muscle and joint tension, massage 1-2 drops to the area of concern. You can also use lemongrass to scare those bugs away by diffusing the oil throughout the affected area or creating your own bug spray. Lastly, you can apply lemongrass topically to support skin health. Simply dilute and rub 1-2 drops softly over the affected area.

General Methods of Application

Apply diluted for sensitive skin. Aromatically. Topically. Internally.

Precautions:

Those with sensitive skin should dilute the oil with a carrier oil. Avoid touching the eyes, ears, and other sensitive areas with the oil. People who are nursing, pregnant, or are receiving medical attention should consult their physician before use. Additionally, make sure to store the oil away from children.

Blend Recipe: DIY Bug Spray

Ingredients:

- 13 drops Cedarwood Essential Oil
- 10 drops Lavender Essential Oil
- 6 drops Eucalyptus Essential Oil
- 5 drops Lemongrass Essential Oil
- 4 drops Peppermint Essential Oil
- 3.5 ounces Distilled Water

Directions:

Do repel mosquitoes or other irritating insects, blend the above ingredients in a 4 ounce glass spray bottle until well mixed. Spray over exposed skin every time you go out of doors.

Lime

Do you wish you had more energy and a brighter attitude? Lime essential oil affects mood with stimulating and refreshing properties

For instance, the oil possesses natural supportive properties when it comes to the immune system. In fact, lime oil can be used aromatically, internally, or topically to fortify the immune system against environmental factors.

The oil refreshes and stimulates the mood and mind, promoting balance and overall wellness. The oil's strong collective properties, along with its natural ability to uplift, make it one powerful agent to have on hand when you're in need of an immune or mental stimulant.

Uses:

To give the mood a pick-me-up, add 3-4 drops lime oil to your diffuser. Sit back and inhale deeply. You can also use lime to clean tough grease or residue from stickers by applying a few drops to a cotton pad and giving it some elbow grease.

For flavoring and internal support, put 1-2 drops into your drinking water and ingest. You can also use lime to promote hair and skin health by placing 1-2 drops in your daily portion of shampoo or facial cleanser.

General Methods of Application

Apply NEAT. Aromatically. Topically.

Precautions:

Those with sensitive skin should dilute the oil with a carrier oil. Avoid touching the eyes, ears, and other sensitive areas with the oil. People who are nursing, pregnant, or are receiving medical attention should consult their physician before use. Additionally, make sure to store the oil away from children. This oil is photosensitive; avoid direct sunlight for 12 hours after applied topically.

Blend Recipe: Limey Hand Sanitizer
Ingredients:

- Distilled Water
- 2 Tbsps Aloe Vera Gel
- 12 drops Lavender Essential Oil
- 8 drops Melaleuca Essential Oil
- 5 drops Lemon Essential Oil
- 5 drops Lime Essential Oil
- 8-10 drops Vitamin E Oil (optional)

Directions:

For a citrusy scented hand sanitizer, combine all ingredients in a glass bottle or container. Fill the remainder with distilled water. Shake vigorously to mix (do this before each use). Apply as needed, rubbing into your hands.

Marjoram

Marjoram is Valued for its calming properties and positive effect on the nervous system. Frequently used by the ancient Greeks and Romans, marjoram oil offers a number of health benefits and is one of your more versatile oils.

For instance, the oil possesses natural calming properties that help support nervous system function. In fact, marjoram can strengthen the function of a number of the body's systems, including the cardiovascular, respiratory, and gastrointestinal systems.

The oil soothes tense muscles, serving as a respite from overwork. Marjoram's strong properties, along with its natural ability to fortify system functions, make it one powerful agent to have on hand when you're facing any health issue.

Uses:

To strengthen respiratory health, add 3-4 drops marjoram and breathe in deeply. For a good night's sleep, you can also diffuse the oil or place a cloth with a drop of marjoram on it near your pillow.

For culinary uses, substitute 1 drop of marjoram essential oil for 2 teaspoons of dried marjoram in any recipe. Lastly, you can apply marjoram topically to support muscle tension. Simply rub 1-2 drops softly over the affected area.

General Methods of Application

Apply NEAT. Aromatically. Internally. Topically.

Precautions:

Those with sensitive skin should dilute the oil with a carrier oil. Avoid touching the eyes, ears, and other sensitive areas with the oil. People who are nursing, pregnant, or are receiving medical attention should consult their physician before use. Additionally, make sure to store the oil away from children.

Blend Recipe: Mild Tension & Head Stress Relief

Ingredients:

- 1 Tbsp Carrier Oil
- 2 drops Lavender Essential Oil
- 2 drops Marjoram Essential Oil
- 1 drop Peppermint Essential Oil

Directions:

Relieve mild tension and stress in the head by blending all oils in a small glass container. Apply topically to the forehead, shoulders, temples, and the back of the neck to soothe and calm tension.

Melaleuca

Often used by the Australian Aborigines, melaleuca oil offers a number of health benefits. For instance, the oil possesses natural cleansing and rejuvenating properties that help fortify the skin, relieving minor skin issues and promoting a clear and younger-looking complexion.

Renowned for its cleansing and rejuvenating effect on the skin, melaleauca oil purifies the air when used with a diffuser.

The oil supplies similar properties when it comes to bodily health by combatting harmful environmental elements and seasonal threats. The oil's strong purifying and cleansing properties, along with its natural ability to support the skin, make it one powerful agent to have on hand when you've got loads of teenagers in the house.

Uses:

To cleanse and purify surfaces or hands, add 3-4 drops melaleuca to a spray bottle then fill the rest with distilled water. Shake well and use as needed.

For bodily health, put 1-2 drops in a veggie capsule and take internally. You can also use melaleuca for a clearer complexion by simply placing a couple drops in your daily cleanser or moisturizer. Lastly, you can apply melaleuca topically to support skin irritations. Simply rub 1-2 drops softly over the affected area.

General Methods of Application

Apply NEAT. Aromatically. Internally. Topically.

Precautions:

Those with sensitive skin should dilute the oil with a carrier oil. Avoid touching the eyes, ears, and other sensitive areas with the oil. People who are nursing, pregnant, or are receiving medical attention should consult their physician before use. Additionally, make sure to store the oil away from children.

Blend Recipe: Lavaleuca Aftershave

Ingredients:

- 1 bottle Fractionated Coconut Oil

- 15 drops Melaleuca Essential Oil
- 15 drops Lavender Essential Oil

Directions:

For a smooth aromatic shave that fortifies skin health, blend all oils in a pump bottle until well combined. Apply the aftershave to the face as normal.

Melissa

Regularly used by the ancient Greeks, melissa oil – or "lemon balm" – offers a number of health benefits. The oil possesses natural digestive properties that help relieve mild stomach discomfort.

In fact, the oil also provides relief from tension and overwrought nerves. Melissa calms the body and eases you into a solid night's sleep. On the other hand, it's quite stimulating when it comes to cognitive function.

The oil's strong immune supportive properties, along with its natural ability to calm and relieve, make it one powerful agent to have on hand when you're in need of comfort.

Uses:

To support digestion and relieve nausea, diffuse or add a couple drops to your hot tea and drink. You can also support the immune system with an internal application or apply 1-2 drops under the tongue.

For emotional health, mix 1-2 drops with a carrier oil and massage into the forehead, chest, and shoulders. You can also use melissa to stimulate cognitive function by using in a room spray. Lastly, you can apply melissa topically to support skin health. Simply rub 1-2 drops softly over the affected area or add to your daily moisturizer.

General Methods of Application

Apply NEAT. Aromatically. Internally. Topically.

Precautions:

Those with sensitive skin should dilute the oil with a carrier oil. Avoid touching the eyes, ears, and other sensitive areas with the oil. People who are nursing, pregnant, or are receiving medical attention should consult their physician before use. Additionally, make sure to store the oil away from children.

Blend Recipe: Massage Oil for Stress Relief
Ingredients:

- 1 Tbsp Carrier Oil
- 1 drop Lavender Essential Oil
- 3 drops Grapefruit Essential Oil
- 3 drops Cinnamon Bark Essential Oil
- 4 drops Roman Chamomile Essential Oil
- 4 drops Fennel Essential Oil
- 5 drops Melissa Essential Oil

Directions:

For a blend of oils that melt away stress and ease achy muscles and joints, blend together the above oils until well combined. Apply in a full-body massage, paying special attention to the neck, back, and shoulders. Recommendation: prior to a stressful event, use this massage blend twice, 6 hours apart.

Myrrh

Myrrh essential oil soothes the skin; promotes a smooth, youthful-looking complexion. Frequently used by the ancients for embalming and religious rituals, myrrh oil offers a number of health benefits.

Myrrh oil possesses natural cleansing properties that help protect against oral decay. In fact, the oil can serve oral health and relieve throat soreness. Myrrh promotes healthier, younger-looking skin by cleansing it and soothing irritations.

The oil's strong cleansing properties, along with its natural ability to strengthen emotional balance, make it one powerful agent to have on hand when you need to put on a happy and radiant face – and smile.

Uses:

Myrrh can cleanse the mouth. To do so, place a couple drops on your toothbrush before adding paste and use as normal. When you combine 1-2 drops myrrh with a small amount of honey and ¼ cup water, you can use the blend to relieve the occasional stomach upset.

Or, consider using myrrh to uplift the mood and promote awareness by diffusing the oil throughout the room. You can also support skin with myrrh by adding 1-2 drops to a moisturizer or lotion.

To cleanse the mouth, add 1-2 drops myrrh to your toothbrush and then apply your toothpaste. Brush your teeth 2-3 times a day.

For emotional health, diffuse throughout the home. You can also blend a couple drops myrrh with ¼ cup water and ½ tsp honey. Take internally to soothe upset stomach. Lastly, you can apply myrrh topically to support skin health. Simply rub 1-2 drops softly over the affected area.

General Methods of Application

Apply NEAT. Aromatically. Internally. Topically.

Precautions:

Those with sensitive skin should dilute the oil with a carrier oil. Avoid touching the eyes, ears, and other sensitive areas with the oil. People who are nursing, pregnant, or are receiving medical attention should consult their physician before use. Additionally, make sure to store the oil away from children.

Blend Recipe: Itchy Foot Relief
Ingredients:

- 2 ounces Carrier Oil
- 6 drops Thyme Essential Oil
- 6 drops Myrrh Essential Oil
- 8 drops Eucalyptus Essential Oil
- 10 drops Tea Tree Essential Oil

Directions:

To relieve occasional itchy feet caused by excess sweat and contamination, blend all ingredients in a small glass container until well combined. Apply 2-3 drops of the blend to the area of concern. Apply two times daily, or as needed. Use consistently and continue two weeks after the issue clears. Store the remainder in a cool, dry place.

Oregano

Oregano essential oil is often used to serve optimal bodily functions. Oregano oil is a "hot" oil that offers a number of health benefits. For instance, the oil possesses high antioxidant content that helps protect against free radicals within the body.

Oregano also offers serious support for digestive issues and helps strengthen respiratory function. The oil combats harmful environmental elements and seasonal threats. The oil's strong purifying and cleansing properties, along with its natural ability to fortify your body's defenses, make it one powerful agent to have on hand during the winter months.

Uses:

To cleanse and purify surfaces, add 3-4 drops oregano to a spray bottle then fill the rest with distilled water. Shake well and use as needed.

For throat soreness, put 1-2 drops in a glass of water and gargle. Substitute a drop into any recipe that calls for oregano. You can also use oregano to fortify the immune system. Dilute with a carrier oil and massage into the body's reflex points or take a drop internally each day.

General Methods of Application

Apply diluted. Aromatically. Topically. Internally.

Precautions:

Those with sensitive skin should dilute the oil with a carrier oil. Avoid touching the eyes, ears, and other sensitive areas with the oil. People who are nursing, pregnant, or are receiving medical attention should consult their physician before use. Additionally, make sure to store the oil away from children.

Blend Recipe: Immune Support Capsule or Massage
Ingredients:

- 5 drops Melissa Essential Oil
- 10 drops Rosemary Essential Oil
- 10 drops Eucalyptus Essential Oil
- 15 drops Oregano Essential Oil
- 15 drops Cinnamon Essential Oil
- 15 drops Black Pepper Essential Oil
- 20 drops Clove Bud Essential Oil
- 30 drops Wild Orange Essential Oil
- 1:1 Coconut Oil (when used externally, dilute)

Directions:

You can use this blend either for immune support externally, internally, or aromatically.

For internal use, add all oils to a 15 mL glass bottle and shake well. Each day after every meal, place 14 drops in a "00" gel capsule and take orally. You can take a single capsule up to three times a day.

For external use, mix 3-5 drops with a carrier oil and massage into the reflex points of the feet.

For aromatic use, diffuse 6-8 drops throughout the home.

Patchouli

Regularly utilized in incense, the scent of patchouli is memorable to those who grew up in the 70's. The oil possesses natural grounding properties that help protect against emotional imbalance.

In fact, reduces the appearance of blemishes, soothes minor skin irritations and promotes a smooth, glowing complexion. The oil stimulates the body's absorption of nutrients, promoting optimal metabolic function and greater energy.

Patchouli's strong skin supportive properties, along with its natural ability to balance emotion, make it one powerful agent to have on hand when you want to look and feel your best.

Uses:

To ground emotions, combine 1-2 drops each of vetiver and patchouli and apply topically to the reflex points, massaging into the skin. For tension relief, massage 1-2 drops into the neck, shoulders, and temples.

You can also apply patchouli topically to support skin health. Simply rub 1-2 drops softly over the affected area.

General Methods of Application

Apply NEAT. Aromatically. Internally. Topically.

Precautions:

Those with sensitive skin should dilute the oil with a carrier oil. Avoid touching the eyes, ears, and other sensitive areas with the oil. People who are nursing, pregnant, or are receiving medical attention should consult their physician before use. Additionally, make sure to store the oil away from children.

Blend Recipe: Aphrodisiac Bath Blend
Ingredients:

- 1-2 Tbsps Sweet Almond Oil
- 1 cup Baking Soda
- 1 cup Refined Salt
- 4 drops Jasmine Essential Oil
- 6 drops Patchouli Essential Oil
- 6 drops Frankincense Essential Oil
- 8 drops Ylang Ylang Essential Oil
- 8 drops Bergamot Essential Oil

Directions:

For an aphrodisiac bath blend, designed to turn up the volume, blend all ingredients in a glass jar. As your hot water is running, place a handful into your bathwater and let disperse. Soak in the sensual and stimulating bath.

Peppermint

Do you suffer from occasional bad breath? Peppermint essential oil is a powerful odor eliminator. A hybrid of spearmint and watermint, peppermint oil offers a number of health benefits.

Peppermint oil possesses natural digestion supportive properties that help relieve minor upsets, like indigestion and nausea. In fact, the oil is also an effective respiratory fortifier, helping clear the airways. Peppermint can be used for oral hygiene, ridding of bad breath and supporting dental health.

This is largely due to its high menthol content. The oil's strong and versatile properties, along with its natural ability to support clear breathing, make it one powerful agent to have on hand when you're short of breath.

Uses:

To support oral health, add 1-2 drops peppermint to a glass of drinking water and take internally. You can also flavor teas, shakes, or baked goods with a single drop of the oil.

For energy or to relieve cravings, inhale peppermint directly. Lastly, you can apply peppermint topically to the stomach or chest to support digestive or respiratory health. Simply dilute 1-2 drops and rub softly over the affected area.

General Methods of Application

Apply diluted for sensitive skin. Aromatically. Topically. Internally.

Precautions:

Those with sensitive skin should dilute the oil with a carrier oil. Avoid touching the eyes, ears, and other sensitive areas with the oil. People who are nursing, pregnant, or are receiving medical attention should consult their physician before use. Additionally, make sure to store the oil away from children.

Blend Recipe: Tired Feet Footbath

Ingredients:

- 1 Tbsp Carrier Oil
- 1 drop Peppermint Essential Oil
- 2 drops Lavender Essential Oil
- 2 drops Geranium Essential Oil

Directions:

For tired and aching feet, treat yourself to an aromatic footbath. Blend all ingredients in a small bowl and add to a basin of hot water. Soak your tired feet for 10-15 minutes.

Roman Chamomile

Does it seem as if your mind is always running a full speed? Even when you try to relax or sleep, you just can't seem to calm the engine.

Roman chamomile will soothe your weary mind. Regularly known as the "plant's physician," Roman chamomile oil offers a number of health benefits. Roman chamomile oil possesses natural calming and soothing properties that help protect against stress and overexertion of the mind, body, and skin.

Roman chamomile can support all systems of the body. The oil strengthens the immune system, supporting overall health and, thereby, defending against environmental hazards. The oil's strong and soothing properties, along with its natural ability to support bodily and mental health, make it one powerful agent to have on hand when your energy is spent.

Uses:

To relax and promote sleep, diffuse Roman chamomile before bedtime or apply topically to the reflex points of the feet. You can also take a couple drops in your hot tea to help you wind down.

For hair and skin support, put 1-2 drops in your shampoo or daily moisturizer and use as normal.

General Methods of Application

Apply NEAT. Aromatically. Internally. Topically.

Precautions:

Those with sensitive skin should dilute the oil with a carrier oil. Avoid touching the eyes, ears, and other sensitive areas with the oil. People who are nursing, pregnant, or are receiving medical attention should consult their physician before use. Additionally, make sure to store the oil away from children.

Blend Recipe: Skin Supportive Salve

Ingredients:

- 2 drops Roman Chamomile Essential Oil
- 2 drops Lavender Essential Oil
- 1 drop Rose Essential Oil
- 1 tsp Grapeseed Oil
- 1 tsp Calendula Oil

Directions:

Support the skin and minor skin irritations with this soothing blend. Blend all ingredients in a small container and apply topically to the area of concern.

Rose

Do scars or blemishes embarrass you? Traditionally used to freshen the skin, rose oil offers a number of health benefits.

For instance, the oil possesses natural hydrating properties that help nourish the skin and protect against dryness. Rose oil reduces the appearance of skin aging and scarring, balances tone and moisture, and enhances the complexion. The oil's strong skin supportive properties, along with its natural ability to uplift, make it one powerful agent to have on hand for your skin.

Uses:

To enhance energy and vitality, add 3-4 drops rose to your diffuser every morning.

For skin health, mix 1-2 drops in with your daily moisturizer and apply as normal. Lastly, you can apply rose directly to support skin health. Simply rub 1-2 drops softly over the affected area.

General Methods of Application

Apply NEAT. Aromatically. Topically.

Precautions:

Those with sensitive skin should dilute the oil with a carrier oil. Avoid touching the eyes, ears, and other sensitive areas with the oil. People who are nursing, pregnant, or are receiving medical attention should consult their physician before use. Additionally, make sure to store the oil away from children.

Blend Recipe: PMS Relief

Ingredients:

- 5 drops Rose Essential Oil
- 5 drops Clary Sage Essential Oil
- 3 drops Bergamot Essential Oil
- 2 ounces Jojoba Oil

Directions:

Relieve PMS with this relaxing blend. Combine all ingredients in a small glass jar or bottle until well blended. Support emotional balance and relieve muscle cramps by massaging over the lower abdomen and the body's reflex points.

Rosemary

Does your stomach make humiliating noises as it turns over in upset? Rosemary supports healthy digestion. Frequently used by the ancient Egyptians, Greeks, and Romans, rosemary offers a number of health benefits.

The oil possesses natural digestive properties that help protect against issues like upset stomach or indigestion. In fact, rosemary can sooth aches and soreness, which makes it an effective oil for muscle and joint health as well.

Moreover, rosemary is a reliever of nervous tension and so can help relieve fatigue. The oil's strong digestive properties, along with its natural ability to flavor, make it one powerful agent to have on hand when you're firing up the summer grill.

Uses:

To strengthen digestion, apply a topical application of rosemary to the abdomen and the reflex points of the feet or add 1-2 drops rosemary to a meat dish or entrée. Not much oil is needed for big flavor.

For emotional support, diffuse the oil throughout the home.

General Methods of Application

Apply NEAT. Aromatically. Internally. Topically.

Precautions:

Those with sensitive skin should dilute the oil with a carrier oil. Avoid touching the eyes, ears, and other sensitive areas with the oil. People who are nursing, pregnant, or are receiving medical attention should consult their physician before use. Additionally, make sure to store the oil away from children.

Blend Recipe: Re-energizing Bath Scrub

Ingredients:

- ¼ cup Avocado Oil
- ½ cup Grapeseed Oil
- ½ cup Epsom Salt
- ½ cup Fine Grain Sea Salt
- 1 Tbsp Vitamin E
- 10 drops Spearmint Essential Oil
- 20 drops Rosemary Essential Oil

Directions:

For an energizing bath scrub, blend the oils in a jar or other airtight container. Blend the salts in a separate container until well combined, then slowly stir them into the oil mixture. Store in a cool, dry place in order to extend the scrub's shelf life. Use as needed.

Sandalwood

Sandalwood oil offers a number of health benefits for your body and mind. For instance, the oil possesses natural grounding properties that help protect against negative emotions.

It is frequently used in meditation to uplift the mind and stimulate the mood. The oil supplies similar properties to skin, making it more radiant, smoother, and healthier than ever.

The oil's strong and calming properties, along with its natural ability to support skin health, make it one powerful agent to have on hand if you have an unwieldy teenager under your roof.

Uses:

To support emotional health and relieve tension, add 3-4 drops to your diffuser and inhale deeply.

For hair health, massage 1-2 drops into your wet hair and scalp. You can also use sandalwood in a facial steam. Add a few drops to a bowl of steaming water, place a towel over it and you, and breathe in the pleasant aroma while the steam goes to work on your pores. Lastly, you can apply sandalwood topically to support skin health. Simply rub 1-2 drops softly over the affected area.

General Methods of Application

Apply NEAT. Aromatically. Internally. Topically.

Precautions:

Those with sensitive skin should dilute the oil with a carrier oil. Avoid touching the eyes, ears, and other sensitive areas with the oil. People who are nursing, pregnant, or are receiving medical attention should consult their physician before use. Additionally, make sure to store the oil away from children.

Blend Recipe: Sultry-scented Body Wash

Ingredients:

- 2/3 cup Liquid Castile Soap
- ¼ cup Honey
- 2 tsps Sweet Almond Oil
- 1 tsp Vitamin E
- 30 drops Ylang Ylang Essential Oil
- 20 drops Sandalwood Essential Oil

Directions:

For a sultry-smelling bath wash, melt the coconut oil over low heat until smooth. Remove the oil from heat and blend in the honey, vitamin E, and essential oils. Whisk until well combined. Slowly add in the castile soap (warning: will suds up, so stir slowly). Once well blended, pour the liquid soap into a glass bottle and shake well. Use as normal. Always shake before use.

Thyme

Does your immune system barely put up a fight? Are you always the first one with a sniffling nose and the last one barely breathing from stuffiness? Thyme will put your defensive line at attention.

Regularly used by the ancient Egyptians and Greeks, thyme oil offers a number of health benefits. Thyme oil possesses natural purifying and cleansing properties that, when applied in small amounts, help promote healthy and clear skin.

The oil utilizes similar properties when it comes to bodily health by combatting harmful environmental elements and seasonal threats. The oil's strong purifying and cleansing properties, along with its natural ability to fortify the immune system, make it one powerful agent to have on hand when your body's in need of a pick-me-up.

Uses:

To support the immune system, add 1-2 drops thyme to a veggie capsule and take internally.

For recipes, put 1 drop in meat or entrees if the herb is called for. Lastly, you can apply thyme topically to support skin health. Simply dilute 1-2 drops and apply gently over the affected area.

General Methods of Application

Apply diluted. Aromatically. Topically. Internally.

Precautions:

Those with sensitive skin should dilute the oil with a carrier oil. Avoid touching the eyes, ears, and other sensitive areas with the oil. People who are nursing, pregnant, or are receiving medical attention should consult their physician before use. Additionally, make sure to store the oil away from children.

Blend Recipe: Poison Ivy Relief

Ingredients:

- 4 Tbsps Carrier Oil
- 2 drops Thyme Essential Oil
- 2 drops Cinnamon Bark Essential Oil
- 13 drops Lemongrass Essential Oil
- 15 drops Rosemary Essential Oil

Directions:

To calm the irritation of poison ivy rash, blend all ingredients together in a small container. Apply over area concern to protect against itching.

Vetiver

Vetiver is used to stabilize emotions and offers a number of health benefits to support the body and mind. The oil possesses natural grounding properties that help protect against emotional issues.

Vetiver can calm the mind, while stimulating healthy blood circulation in the body. The oil strengthens immune system function, thereby supporting the body in protecting against harmful environmental elements and seasonal threats.

The oil's strong stabilizing properties, along with its natural ability to promote immune system function, make it one powerful agent to have on hand when you're dragging through the winter.

Uses:

To strengthen the immune system, add 1-2 drops to your hot tea and ingest. Diffuse the oil with lavender to promote healthy emotional balance

For relaxation, put 1-2 drops in your bathwater and soak. You can also use vetiver to promote healthy circulation by using it in a massage. You only need a tiny amount of vetiver to get the full effect of its health benefits, so consider applying with a toothpick.

General Methods of Application

Apply NEAT. Aromatically. Internally. Topically.

Precautions:

Those with sensitive skin should dilute the oil with a carrier oil. Avoid touching the eyes, ears, and other sensitive areas with the oil. People who are nursing, pregnant, or are receiving medical attention should consult their physician before use. Additionally, make sure to store the oil away from children.

Blend Recipe: Vetiver Body Butter

Ingredients:

- ½ cup Shea Butter
- ¼ cup Almond Oil

- ¼ cup Coconut Oil (solid)
- 8 drops Vetiver Essential Oil
- 8 drops Jasmine Essential Oil

Directions:

For a smooth, skin supportive body butter, melt the shea butter and coconut oil in a pan over medium low heat. Stir until smooth and well combined. Remove the mixture from the stove and stir in the remaining oils. Scoop the body butter into a glass container with a tight lid. Use a small amount over the elbows, feet, cuticles, and other dry areas of the body.

White Fir

Do you feel as though Christmas is a hassle? Do you imagine you're destined to be the Grinch or Scrooge of the holidays? Well, start spreading the cheer with the scent of white fir to lift your spirits!

A common holiday fragrance, white fir oil offers a number of health benefits. For instance, the oil possesses natural soothing properties that help relieve sore muscles and joints and enable relaxation. In fact, white fir also soothes respiratory issues, supporting clear breathing and overall respiratory function.

White Fir oil stabilizes, empowers, and energizes the mind and body. The oil's strong and soothing properties, along with its natural ability to support the respiratory tract, make it one powerful agent to have on hand when your body is in need of relief.

Uses:

To fortify respiratory function, apply white fir topically to the chest or diffuse it throughout your home.

For relaxation and sore muscle relief, put 1-2 drops in your bathwater. You can also use white fir to stimulate cognitive function and relieve mental fatigue by breathing the aroma in, directly.

General Methods of Application

Apply NEAT. Aromatically. Topically.

Precautions:

Those with sensitive skin should dilute the oil with a carrier oil. Avoid touching the eyes, ears, and other sensitive areas with the oil. People who are nursing, pregnant, or are receiving medical attention should consult their physician before use. Additionally, make sure to store the oil away from children.

Blend Recipe: Muscle & Joint Relief
Ingredients:

- 30 drops White Fir Essential Oil
- 10 drops Helichrysum Essential Oil
- 5 drops Peppermint Essential Oil
- 1 drop Oregano Essential Oil
- 3 ounces Carrier Oil

Directions:

Relieve muscle or arthritic aches and pains by blending all oils together in a small glass jar. Shake well and apply to the affected area, massaging gently over arthritic knees or wrists or aching muscles.

Wild Orange

A popular oil for cleaning and freshening, wild orange oil also offers a number of health benefits. For instance, the oil possesses a high level of antioxidants which helps combat those harmful free radicals within the body.

Wild orange can even be used as a surface disinfectant for tabletops, dishes, floors, and anything in between. The oil supplies similar properties when it comes to bodily health by combatting harmful environmental elements and seasonal threats.

The oil's strong purifying and cleansing properties, along with its natural ability to disinfect, make it one powerful agent to have on hand for Spring cleaning.

Uses:

To cleanse and purify surfaces, add 3-4 drops wild orange to a spray bottle then fill the rest with distilled water. Shake well and use as needed.

For flavor and health benefits, put 1-2 drops of wild orange in a glass of drinking water. You can also use the oil aromatically by diffusing throughout the room. Lastly, you can apply the cup and inhale method to boost energy.

General Methods of Application

Apply NEAT. Aromatically. Internally. Topically.

Precautions:

Those with sensitive skin should dilute the oil with a carrier oil. Avoid touching the eyes, ears, and other sensitive areas with the oil. People who are nursing, pregnant, or are receiving medical attention should consult their physician before use. Additionally, make sure to store the oil away from children. This oil is photosensitive; avoid direct sunlight for 12 hours after applied topically.

Blend Recipe: Wild Geranium Massage
Ingredients:
- 15 mL Carrier Oil

- 10 drops Geranium Essential Oil
- 5 drops Wild Orange Essential Oil

Directions:

Relieve nerves and stress while melting away muscle soreness with this massage blend. In a small glass jar or bottle, add all ingredients and shake well to mix. Massage into the neck, feet, shoulders, and lower back.

Wintergreen

Do irregular breathing patterns keep you up at night? Wintergreen oil will open up your airways, enabling a much more restful sleep. Often used to flavor gums and toothpastes, wintergreen oil comes from a low-growing shrub and offers a number of health benefits.

Wintergreen oil possesses natural soothing properties that help support aching muscles and joints. In fact, the oil also supports respiratory health, clearing airways and promoting breathing. Although the oil is too powerful to be taken internally, it does serve as a flavoring for many oral products.

The oil's strong properties, along with its natural ability to support respiratory function, make it one powerful agent to have on hand during the winter months.

Uses:

To alleviate sore muscles and achy joints, dilute 1-2 drops wintergreen and apply it to the problem areas. For a bath time muscle-melting soak, place 1-2 drops in your running bathwater to disperse, and sink in to delectable comfort.

General Methods of Application

Apply diluted for sensitive skin. Aromatically. Topically.

Precautions:

Those with sensitive skin should dilute the oil with a carrier oil. Avoid touching the eyes, ears, and other sensitive areas with the oil. People who are nursing, pregnant, or are receiving medical attention should consult their physician before use. Additionally, make sure to store the oil away from children.

Blend Recipe: Head Tension & Stress Relief
Ingredients:

- 4 tsps Carrier Oil
- 5 drops Clove Essential Oil
- 6 drops Ginger Essential Oil
- 9 drops Wintergreen Essential Oil
- 9 drops Peppermint Essential Oil

Directions:

Ease tension and stress in the head by blending all ingredients in a small glass jar or bottle. Apply topically to the forehead, temples, shoulders, back of the neck, and into the body's reflex points.

Ylang Ylang

Regularly utilized in perfumes and aromatherapy, ylang ylang oil offers a number of health benefits for the body and mind. For instance, the oil possesses natural skin-fortifying properties that support the skin and hair.

Ylang Ylang oil supports hormonal balance, which serves the skin, emotions, and hormonal fluctuation during menopause and menstruation. The oil serves mental and emotional health by calming tension and stress and prompting a positive outlook. The oil's strong supportive properties, along with its natural ability to enhance the skin, make it one powerful agent to have on hand when you're hormones are in flux.

Uses:

To promote relaxation, add 3-4 drops ylang ylang to your bathwater. Soak and inhale slowly and deeply for twenty minutes. Afterwards, you can apply ylang ylang on your pulse points, neck, and wrists to use as a perfume.

Lastly, you can apply ylang ylang topically to support skin health. Simply rub 1-2 drops softly over the affected area.

General Methods of Application

Apply NEAT. Aromatically. Internally. Topically.

Precautions:

Those with sensitive skin should dilute the oil with a carrier oil. Avoid touching the eyes, ears, and other sensitive areas with

the oil. People who are nursing, pregnant, or are receiving medical attention should consult their physician before use. Additionally, make sure to store the oil away from children.

Blend Recipe: Male Libido Stimulant

Ingredients:

- 3-4 drops Ylang Ylang
- 3-4 drops Clary Sage

Directions:

Stimulate male libido by adding the oils to a "00" capsule. Take a single capsule, twice daily after meals.